A RELIABLE AND ACCURATE HEART DISEASE PREDICTION SYSTEM

by

G. PURUSOTHAMAN

ABSTRACT

Heart disease has increased quickly by reason of varying lifestyle combined with improper or lack of physical exercise, foretelling and averting the heart diseases at prior stage has turn out to be a significant action as in every year root to death. Plentiful researchers presented in the current work for health disease prediction.

In the first work, initially Pre-processing is done by using K-means clustering Algorithm to make the dataset cleaner, consistent and noise free. Then Feature reduction of the dataset is done by using Fuzzy based rough set theory. The fuzzy rough sets extend the rough set concept through the use of fuzzy equivalence classes. From this reduced feature set, optimal feature selection is done by using Improved Bee Colony approach. Finally, classification of dataset is done by using Support vector machine. The overall evaluation of the proposed research methodology is done by using the Matlab simulation environment from which it is proved that the proposed work namely NORFS-HDPS can lead to optimal outcome than the existing research techniques.

In the second work introducing the framework namely Heart disease prediction using Alpha Rough Set Theory combined with Fuzzy SVM (ARST-FSVM). In this research method, Modified K-Means clustering algorithm is used for preprocessing the input dataset which would avoid the noisy data present in the database. Then missing data value in the database is handled using normalization technique where NLLS imputation is applied. And then feature dimensionality reduction is done using Alpha rough set theory (α-RST) approach. From those reduced feature set, optimal feature selection in terms of relevancy is done using Hybrid Bee colony algorithm with Glowworm Swarm Optimization (HBC-GSO) approach. Finally heart disease prediction is done using classifier namely fuzzy based SVM. The overall research method ensures that the proposed research technique leads to ensure it can lead to optimal and accurate heart disease diagnosis outcome.

In the third work introducing the Accurate and reliable heart disease prediction with the concern of Risk factors using Hybrid Rough Set-Hybrid Multi Class SVM (HRS-HMCSVM). The proposed research method can optimally predict the heart disease occurrence earlier with increased prediction accuracy. In this research method Hybrid K-

Means clustering algorithm is applied to preprocess the dataset. After preprocessing, missing value replacement is done by using imputation methods. And then dimensionality reduction is done by using Hybrid Rough set theory concept which is sent to feature selection module where the optimal features are extracted by using Hybrid Improved Bee Colony with Cuckoo Search Algorithm. Finally, Classification of the dataset is done using Fuzzy SVM approach.

The overall evaluation of the research method is conducted in the mat lab simulation environment under heart disease sample dataset gathered from the multiple users. This comparison evaluation proves that the proposed research method leads to provide the optimal outcome than the existing research techniques.

TABLE OF CONTENTS

LIST OF FIGURES

LIST OF TABLES

LIST OF ABBREVIATIONS

CVD	Cardio Vascular Disease
ACE	Angiotensin Converting Enzyme
KDD	Knowledge Discovery in Databases
CART	Classification and Regression Trees
CHAID	Chi Square Automatic Interaction Detection
EDA	Exploratory Data Analysis
CDA	Confirmatory Data Analysis
NORFS-HDPS	Noise aware Optimal Risk Factor Selection for Heart Disease Prediction System
ARST-FSVM	Alpha Rough Set Theory combined with Fuzzy SVM
HRS-HMCSVM	Hybrid Rough Set-Hybrid Multi Class SVM
CNN	Convolutional Neural Network
AUC	Area Under the ROC Curve
RGB	Red Green Blue
CSN-I	Color Space Normalized-I
PCA	Principal Component Analysis
APGL	Accelerated Proximal Gradient algorithm
IEHPS	Intelligent and Effective Heart Attack Prediction
FIM	Frequent Itemset Mining
MAFIA	MAximal Frequent Itemset Algorithm
MCECM	Multi-Cycle Expectation Conditional Maximization
HDL	High Density Lipoprotein cholesterol
BMI	Body Mass Index
ECG	ElectroCardioGram
FD	Fractal Dimension
H	Hurst's exponent
DFA	Detrended Fluctuation Analysis
ApproxEnt	Approximate Entropy

SampEnt	Sample Entropy
CD	Correlation Dimension
DWT	Discrete Wavelet Transform
SCDI	Sudden Cardiac Death Index
DT	Decision Tree
KNN	k-Nearest Neighbour
SVM	Support Vector Machine
PSO	Particle Swarm Optimization
PSO-RR	PSO based Relative Reduct
PSO-QR	PSO based Quick Reduct
SVM-REF	Support Vector Machines Recursive Feature Elimination
BDF	Binary Dragon Fly
CT	Computed Tomography
RECIST	Response Evaluation Criteria in Solid Tumors
GALA	Genetic Algorithm and Learning Automata
SSO	Social Spider Optimization
GA	Genetic Algorithm
CBFA	Cooperative Bacterial Foraging Algorithm
AFSO	Artificial Fish Swarm Optimization
ACO/PSO	Ant Colony Optimization/Particle Swarm Optimization
ROI	Region Of Interest
FCBF	Fast Correlation-Based Filter solution
BBBO	Binary Biogeography Based Optimization
MOBBBO	Multi-Objective Binary Biogeography Based Optimization
LOOCV	Leave-One-Out Cross-Validation method
MLP	Multi-Layer Perceptron
HPLC-LIF	High Performance Liquid Chromatography-Laser Induced Fluorescence
SVR	Support Vector Regression
ELM	Extreme Learning Machine

MARS	Multivariate Adaptive Regression Splines
RF	Random Forest
FIGO	International Federation of Gynecology and Obstetrics
ALH	Adaptive Local Hyperplane
MVE	Missing Value Estimation
GRNN	Generalized Regression Neural Network
GLCM	Grey Level Co-occurrence Matrices
FNN	Fuzzy Neural Network
LDA	Linear Discriminant Analysis
BDLDA	Block Diagonal Linear Discriminant Analysis
ABC	Artificial bee colony
CHD-PSO	Coronary Heart Disease prediction using Particle Swarm Optimization Approach
ANN	Artificial Neural Network
α-RST	Alpha rough set theory
HBC-GSO	Hybrid Bee colony algorithm with Glowworm Swarm Optimization
KM	K-Means
MICE	Multiple Imputation by Chained Equations
NLLS	New Local Least Square imputation
GSO	Glow Worm Swarm Optimization
WHO	World Health Organization
BP	Blood Pressure
RMSE	Root Mean Square Error
FIML	Full Information Maximum Likelihood

CHAPTER 1

INTRODUCTION

Data mining has already established as a novel field for exploring hidden patterns in the huge datasets (Witten et al., 2016). Medical science is another field where large amount of data is generated using different clinical reports and other patient symptoms. Data mining can also be used heavily for the same purpose in medical datasets also. These explored hidden patterns in medical datasets can be used for clinical diagnosis. However, medical datasets are widely dispersed, heterogeneous, and huge in nature. These datasets need to be organized and integrated with the hospital management systems (Ristoski, and Paulheim, 2016).

Cardiovascular diseases are one of the highest flying diseases of the modern world. According to world health organization about more than 12 million deaths occurs worldwide, every year due to heart problems (Shah et al., 2015). It is also one of the fatal diseases in India which causes maximum casualties. The diagnosis of this disease is intricate process. It should be diagnosed accurately and correctly. Due to limitation of the potential of the medical experts and their unavailability at certain places put their patients at high risk. Normally, it is diagnosed using intuition of the medical specialist (Sultan, 2015). It would be highly advantageous if the techniques will be integrated with the medical information system. A computer based information or decision support systems can facilitate accurate diagnosis that's too at reduced cost. This integration of varied data mining techniques with the existing medical decision support system requires comparison of different data mining techniques for finding out their suitability for the said job.

1.1. INTRODUCTION ABOUT HEART DISEASE

Heart disease or cardiovascular disease is the class of diseases that involve the heart or blood vessels (arteries and veins) (Dawber et al., 2015). Today most countries face high and increasing rates of heart disease and it has become a leading cause of debilitation and death worldwide in men and women over age sixty-five and today in many countries heart disease is viewed as a "second epidemic," replacing infectious diseases as the leading cause of death. Traditionally, heart disease was thought to be the problem of developed countries, but now it is becoming a headache for developing countries too and it is especially devastating for the developing countries since they do not have adequate health care (Patel and Sharma, 2015). As noted by Office on Women's Health heart disease was considered to be a man's problem, but now it is recognized as number one killer of women, just as it is of men.

Making a diagnosis of heart disease includes taking a complete medical evaluation and history and physical examination and early diagnosis of heart disease can help reduce the rate of mortality (McCrindle et al., 2017). One of the best ways to diagnose a heart disease is by using echocardiography. Echocardiography, or echo, is a painless test that uses sound waves to create pictures of the heart. The test gives information about the size and shape of the heart and how well the heart chambers and valves are working. Echo also can be done to detect heart problems in infants and children. The test also can identify areas of heart muscle that aren't contracting normally due to poor blood flow or injury from a previous heart attack (Allan et al., 2018). In addition, a type of echo called Doppler ultrasound shows how well blood flows through the chambers and valves of the heart.

As described by National Heart Lung and Blood Institute echo can detect possible blood clots inside the heart, fluid buildup in the pericardium (the sac around the heart), and problems with the aorta (aorta is the main artery that carries oxygen-rich blood from the heart to the body) (Nichols et al., 2015). But, the interpretation of echo recordings remains a challenge since there are no available precise rules that are deduced from databases. The analysis of Echo data by experts is time consuming and this is in concomitant with the shortage of experts possessing knowledge on the analysis of Echo data (Wang et al., 2016). Thus, methods to automate the interpretation of Echo recordings by minimizing human efforts are important for diagnosis of heart disease in patients. In order to solve this and many other problems in the health sector related to disease diagnosis, one has to come up with a way to extract hidden information from enormous datasets that are collected in the past. Data mining can be a solution by generating rules from those enormous datasets which can be used in echo readings (Shmueli et al., 2017). Cardio Vascular Disease (CVD) is a general term for a disease of the heart or blood vessels.

Blood flow to the heart, brain or body is reduced because of:

- a blood clot (thrombosis)
- a build-up of fatty deposits inside an artery, leading to hardening and narrowing of the artery (atherosclerosis)

Types of CVD are listed as follows:

The three main types of CVD are:

- coronary heart disease
- stroke
- peripheral arterial disease

1.1.1. Coronary Heart Disease

Coronary heart disease occurs when your heart's blood supply is blocked or interrupted by a build-up of fatty substances (called atheroma) in the coronary arteries (Council, 2017). The coronary arteries are two major blood vessels that supply the heart with blood. If your coronary arteries become narrow due to a build-up of atheroma, the blood supply to your heart will be restricted. This can cause angina (chest pains). If a coronary artery becomes completely blocked, it can cause a heart attack.

1.1.2. Stroke

A stroke is a serious medical condition that occurs when the blood supply to the brain is disturbed (Kalladka et al., 2016). Like all organs, your brain needs oxygen and nutrients provided by the blood to function properly. If the supply of blood is restricted or stopped, brain cells begin to die. This can lead to brain damage and possibly death. A stroke is a medical emergency. Prompt treatment is essential because the sooner a person receives treatment for a stroke, the less damage is likely to happen. There are two main types of stroke:

- ischemic (accounting for 70% of all strokes): the blood supply is stopped due to a blood clot
- hemorrhagic: a weakened blood vessel supplying the brain bursts and causes brain damage

1.1.3. Peripheral Arterial Disease

Peripheral arterial disease, also known as peripheral vascular disease, occurs when there is a blockage in the arteries to your limbs (usually your legs) (Greaves, 2017). The most common symptom of peripheral arterial disease is pain in your legs. This is usually in one or both of your thighs, hips or calves. The pain can feel like a cramp, a dull pain or a sensation of heaviness in the muscles of your legs. It usually comes and goes, and gets worse during exercise that uses your legs, such as walking or climbing stairs.

1.1.4. Impact on Public Health

CVD is the leading cause of death in Ireland and worldwide (Bhatnagar et al., 2015). In 2010, one-third of all deaths in Ireland (9,182 deaths) were due to CVD. Of these deaths:

- 4,625 were caused by coronary heart disease
- 2,015 were caused by stroke

It is thought that most deaths due to CVD are premature and could be prevented by making a number of lifestyle changes It is estimated that CVD is responsible for around one in three premature deaths in men and one in five premature deaths in women.

1.2. RISK FACTORS OF HEART DISEASE PREDICTION SYSTEM

Risk factors are variables that predict who is most likely to develop CVD (McClelland et al., 2015). Most of the risk factors for cardiovascular disease and stroke are modifiable or entirely preventable. By modifying risk factors, you decrease the chances of getting diseases. Modifiable risk factors include tobacco use, high blood pressure, physical inactivity, high blood cholesterol, obesity, heavy alcohol consumption, and poor nutrition. Non-modifiable risk factors are age and family history. The more risk factors one has, the higher the risk of developing disease. Understanding these risk factors is crucial to achieving optimal heart health.

Here are the 5 main risk factors for heart disease:

1. Hypertension (high blood pressure)

2. Diabetes mellitus

3. High cholesterol

4. Tobacco use

5. Genetics

Every person is born with healthy arteries. Over time, factors from our diet and lifestyle can damage the lining of the arteries called the "endothelium." When the endothelium is injured, it becomes inflamed and eventually cholesterol sticks in the wall of the arteries. The process by which this cholesterol plaque builds up is called "atherosclerosis." Look at these 5 risk factors. We can directly prevent 4 of the 5 with lifestyle changes. Genetics are out of our control sort of, but as you will see your lifestyle choices actually do affect if you express genes leading to heart disease (Osborn et al., 2015). Thus, even if heart disease "runs in the family", you are not destined to get heart disease if you make the correct lifestyle changes. Controlling all the risk factors that we can by healthy lifestyle living can essentially prevent atherosclerosis from occurring in any part of your body and even reverse it in many cases. Each of these risk factors will have their own video, but here that are briefly.

1.2.1. Hypertension

Hypertension is present when the pressure inside the arteries is higher than it should be. This puts too much stress by sheer force on the wall of the arteries and the endothelium leading to damage and eventually cholesterol plaque build-up (Parati et al., 2014). The high pressure can also lead to aneurysm formation in an artery and even rupture which can be life threatening. Risk factors of hyper tension is shown in the following figure 1.1.

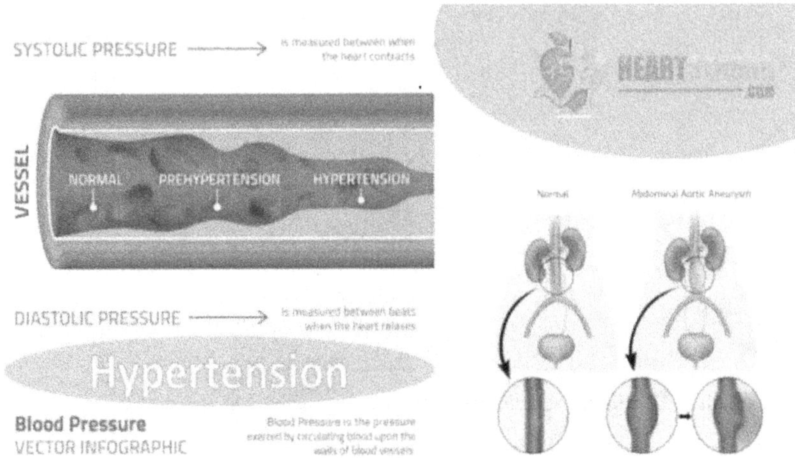

Figure 1.1. Hypertension Risk Factor

1.2.2. Diabetes Mellitus

Diabetes mellitus comes in two types: Type I and Type II (Asmat et al., 2016). Type I diabetes frequently occurs in childhood and is the result of an organ called the pancreas not producing the glucose lowering hormone insulin. Type II diabetes is the form that is from "insulin resistance." This is the type that is predominately caused by poor dietary habits, obesity and lack of physical activity.

1.2.3. High Cholesterol

The causes and flow of high cholesterol occurrence is shown in the following figure 1.2.

Cholesterol is a fatty substance important for the function of all cells (Vinarova et al., 2015). What many do not realized is that cholesterol is made in your liver.

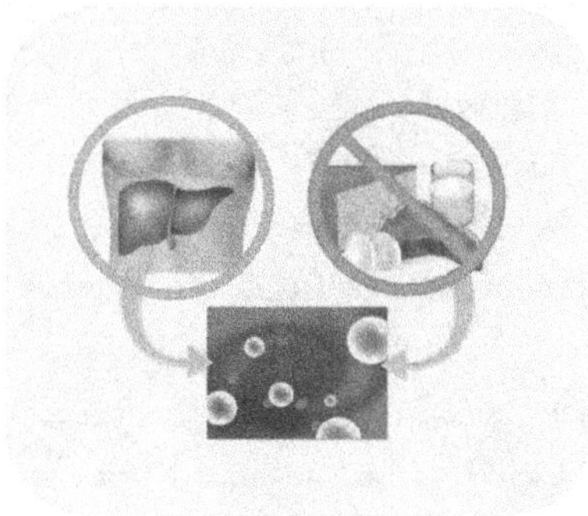

Figure 1.2. Causes and flow of High Cholesterol

You DO NOT need to eat any cholesterol to survive. Having high levels of cholesterol in the blood significantly worsens the atherosclerotic processes increasing the risk of heart attack and stroke. Cholesterol in the diet is ONLY found in animal products such as meat, dairy and eggs. There is NO cholesterol in any plant product.

1.2.4. Tobacco Use

Smoking tobacco products introduces multiple toxins into the system which has many negative health effects (Grana et al., 2014). One of these effects is damage to the endothelial cells. Any damage to the endothelium, as you have learned, can speed up the harmful process of atherosclerosis. Cholesterol formation and blood vessel blockage happening due to tobacco use is shown in the following figure 1.3.

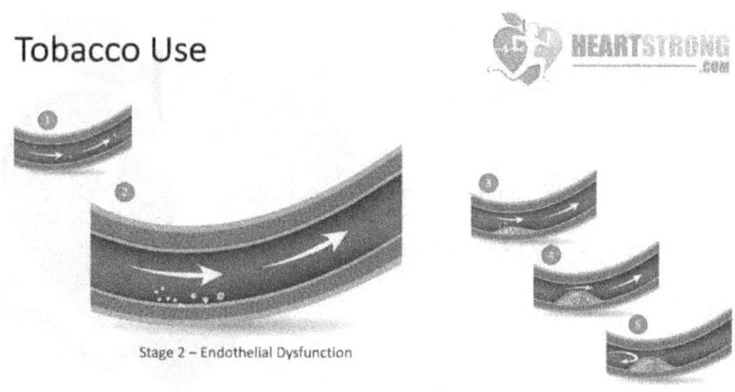

Figure 1.3. Results of Tobacco use

1.2.5. Genetics

Many people think genetics play a large role in heart disease development (Soininen et al., 2015). This is actually not the case. Families in which heart disease strikes at a younger age frequently have unhealthy lifestyle habits in common such as diets high in cholesterol and saturated fat, lack of physical activity and the use of tobacco products. It is now known the exact percentage of heart disease that is purely genetic, but estimates say that at least 90% of heart disease is preventable. Many experts think 99% of heart disease is preventable. If this is the case then 1% or less of heart disease would be purely genetic. What is largely unknown is how much strict lifestyle changes including a whole foods plant based diet will lower the risk of people who adopt this eating pattern at a young age along with avoiding toxins like tobacco and staying physically active.

1.3. PREVENTING CARDIOVASCULAR DISEASE IN ADULTS

Most of the factors that increase your risk of CVD are linked (Fox et al., 2015). This means that if you have one of these risk factors, you will probably have others as well. For example, people who drink alcohol heavily usually have poor diets and are more likely to smoke. Obese people are more likely to have diabetes, high cholesterol and high blood pressure. Addressing one risk factor (such as quitting smoking) will bring important health benefits, but to achieve a significant reduction in your CVD risk, you need to look at your lifestyle as a whole. In particular, you need to consider (Bibbins-Domingo et al., 2016):

- the amount of alcohol you drink
- your diet
- your weight
- how much exercise and physical activity you do
- whether you need to stop smoking

1.3.1. Alcohol

If you drink alcohol, do not exceed the recommended daily limits of three to four units a day for men and two to three units a day for women. A unit of alcohol is roughly half a pint of normal strength lager, a small glass of wine or a single measure of spirits. Counseling services and medication can help you reduce your alcohol intake.

1.3.2. Diet

A low-fat, high-fibre diet that includes whole grains and plenty of fresh fruit and vegetables (at least five portions a day) is recommended for a healthy heart. Limit the amount of salt in your diet to no more than 6g (0.2oz or 1 teaspoon) a day. Too much salt will increase your blood pressure. Do not eat foods that are high in saturated fat because this will increase your cholesterol level.

These include: "meat pies, sausages and fatty cuts of meat, butter, ghee (a type of butter often used in Indian cooking), lard, cream, hard cheese, cakes and biscuits, foods that contain coconut or palm oil". Eating some foods that are high in unsaturated fat can help decrease your cholesterol level. These foods include: "oily fish, avocados, nuts and seeds, sunflower oil, rapeseed, olive oil".

1.3.3. Weight Management

If you are overweight or obese, you can lose weight and maintain a healthy weight with a combination of regular exercise and a calorie-controlled diet.

1.3.4. Regular Exercise

It is recommended that adults should do at least 150 minutes (2 hours and 30 minutes) of moderate-intensity aerobic activity (i.e. cycling or fast walking) every week. Activities you could incorporate into your exercise programme include: "brisk walking, hill climbing, running, cycling, swimming".

If you find it difficult to do 150 minutes of moderate-intensity exercise each week, start at a level you feel comfortable with. For example, do five to ten minutes of light exercise a day and gradually increase the duration and intensity of your activity as your fitness level improves.

1.3.5. Medications

If your risk of developing CVD is thought to be particularly high, you may be prescribed medication to reduce your risk. Medications used to prevent CVD include:

"statins, which are used to lower blood cholesterol levels, anticoagulants (such as warfarin or low-dose aspirin), which are used to prevent blood clots, Angiotensin Converting Enzyme (ACE) inhibitors, which are used to treat high blood pressure".

1.4. PREVENTING CARDIOVASCULAR DISEASE IN CHILDREN

There is a lot of good-quality evidence that eating and drinking habits established during childhood can continue for many years into adulthood (Yusuf et al., 2015). So while bad eating habits in childhood may not pose an immediate health risk, they could lead to serious health problems in adulthood. Four important things to consider are: "the amount of salt your child eats, how much fat they eat, how much sugar they eat, the amount of exercise they do.

1.4.1. Salt

Eating high levels of salt in childhood has been linked to an increased risk of high blood pressure, heart disease and stroke in adulthood. The current recommended limits of salt for children are: "for children aged 0-6 months: less than 1g of salt a day, for children aged 7-12 months: 1g a day, for children aged 1-3 years: 2g a day, for children aged 4-6 years: 3g a day, for children aged 7-10 years: 5g a day, for children aged 11-14 years: 6g a day". It is easy to underestimate how much salt is contained in food. For example, a Happy Meal containing small fries, a hamburger and a coke contains 1.8g of salt, which is over half the recommended daily limit for a five-year-old. Pre-packaged and ready-to-eat foods (especially those not specifically designed for children) contain high levels of salt. For example, a 200g tin of tomato soup contains 1.4g of salt. Check the label of any foods you give your child so you can keep an eye on their daily salt consumption.

1.4.2. Fats and Sugar

Limit the amount of saturated fat and sugar your child eats. Too much of these can lead to high cholesterol, diabetes and high blood pressure in later life. They can also increase your child's risk of becoming overweight or obese, and a diet high in sugar can cause tooth decay. Children's foods that are high in saturated fats and sugar include: "chocolate, sweets, fast food such as burgers or chicken nuggets, fizzy drinks, ice cream, biscuits, crisps, processed foods, such as microwave meals, hot dogs and breakfast cereals that contain additional sugar".

1.4.3. Exercise

Most children are naturally active and full of energy. However, as many of today's pastimes are inactive, such as watching TV and playing computer games, many children do not get the exercise they need. It is now recommended that:

- Children (under 5 years) who can walk unaided should be physically active every day for at least 180 minutes (3 hours), spread throughout the day, indoors or out.
- Children and young people (5 to 18 years) should do at least 60 minutes (1 hour) of aerobic activity every day, which should include a mix of moderate-intensity (i.e. fast walking) and vigorous-intensity (i.e. running) activities.

This amount of exercise is enough to strengthen bones and muscles and can help prevent children putting on weight. There are many different ways for children to exercise. Simply walking or cycling to school is a good way to start. Team sports can also be great fun and can improve co-ordination, balance and team skills. Most community sports centers run team activities for children, such as football, basketball and volleyball. Ask your local sports centre for more information. If your children do not like team sports, there are plenty of other fun activities for them to try, such as swimming, dance and martial arts.

1.5. DATA MINING IN HEART DISEASE PREDICTION

Data mining is a crucial step in discovery of knowledge from large datasets. In recent years, Data mining has found its significant hold in every field including health care. Mining process is more than the data analysis which includes classification, clustering, and association rule discovery. It also spans other disciplines like Data Warehousing, Statistics, Machine learning and Artificial Intelligence. Data mining is predicted to be one of the most revolutionary developments of the century, according to the online technology magazine ZDNET News. In fact, The Technology Review Ten, chose data mining as one of 10 emerging technologies that will change the world. Effectively analyzing information from customers, partners, and suppliers has become important to more companies. Furthermore, many companies have implemented a data warehouse strategy and are now starting to look at what they can do with all that data.

Data mining can be a useful tool in the health sector and healthcare (Wang et al., 2018). Organizations that perform data mining are better positioned to meet their long-term needs, many authors argued that data can be a great asset to healthcare organizations, but they have to be first transformed into information. Predicting the outcome of a disease is one of the most interesting and challenging tasks in which to develop data mining applications. In recent years new research avenues such as Knowledge Discovery in Databases (KDD), which includes data mining techniques, has become a popular research tool for medical researchers who seek to identify and exploit patterns and relationships among large number of variables, and be able to predict the outcome of a disease using the historical cases stored within datasets.

The healthcare industry collects large amounts of health-care data and that need to be mined to discover hidden information for effective decision making. Motivated by the world-wide increasing mortality of heart disease patients each year and the availability of huge amount of patients' data from which to extract useful knowledge, researchers have been using data mining techniques to help health care professionals in the diagnosis of heart disease. Data mining is the exploration of large datasets to extract hidden and previously unknown patterns, relationships and knowledge that are difficult to detect with traditional statistical methods. Thus data mining refers to mining or extracting knowledge from large amounts of data. Data mining applications will be used for better health policy-making and prevention of hospital errors, early detection, prevention of diseases and preventable hospital deaths. Heart disease prediction system can assist medical professionals in predicting heart disease based on the clinical data of patients. Hence by implementing a heart disease prediction system using Data Mining techniques and doing some sort of data mining on various heart disease attributes, it can able to predict more probabilistically that the patients will be diagnosed with heart disease.

1.6. DATA MINING

Data mining, the extraction of hidden predictive information from large databases, is a powerful new technology with great potential to help companies focus on the most important information in their data warehouses (Thomas et al., 2017). Data mining tools predict future trends and behaviors, allowing businesses to make proactive, knowledge-driven decisions. The automated, prospective analyses offered by data mining move beyond the analyses of past events provided by retrospective tools typical of decision support systems. Data mining tools can answer business questions that traditionally were too time consuming to resolve. They scour databases for hidden patterns, finding predictive information that experts may miss because it lies outside their expectations. Most companies already collect and refine massive quantities of data. Data mining techniques can be implemented rapidly on existing software and hardware platforms to enhance the value of existing information resources, and can be integrated with new products and systems as they are brought on-line.

1.6.1. The Scope of Data Mining

Data mining derives its name from the similarities between searching for valuable business information in a large database for example, finding linked products in gigabytes of store scanner data and mining a mountain for a vein of valuable ore. Both processes require either sifting through an immense amount of material, or intelligently probing it to find exactly where the value resides. Given databases of sufficient size and quality, data mining technology can generate new business opportunities by providing these capabilities (Jain et al., 2017):

- **Automated prediction of trends and behaviors**. Data mining automates the process of finding predictive information in large databases. Questions that traditionally required extensive hands-on analysis can now be answered directly from the data quickly. A typical example of a predictive problem is targeted marketing. Data mining uses data on past promotional mailings to identify the targets most likely to maximize return on investment in future mailings. Other predictive problems include forecasting bankruptcy and other forms of default, and identifying segments of a population likely to respond similarly to given events.
- **Automated discovery of previously unknown patterns**. Data mining tools sweep through databases and identify previously hidden patterns in one step. An example of pattern discovery is the analysis of retail sales data to identify seemingly unrelated products that are often purchased together. Other pattern discovery problems include detecting fraudulent credit card transactions and identifying anomalous data that could represent data entry keying errors.

Data mining techniques can yield the benefits of automation on existing software and hardware platforms, and can be implemented on new systems as existing platforms are upgraded and new products developed. When data mining tools are implemented on high performance parallel processing systems, they can analyze massive databases in minutes. Faster processing means that users can automatically experiment with more models to understand complex data. High speed makes it practical for users to analyze huge quantities of data. Larger databases, in turn, yield improved predictions. Databases can be larger in both depth and breadth:

- **More columns**. Analysts must often limit the number of variables they examine when doing hands-on analysis due to time constraints. Yet variables that are discarded because they seem unimportant may carry information about unknown patterns. High performance data mining allows users to explore the full depth of a database, without preselecting a subset of variables.
- **More rows**. Larger samples yield lower estimation errors and variance, and allow users to make inferences about small but important segments of a population.

A recent Gartner Group Advanced Technology Research Note listed data mining and artificial intelligence at the top of the five key technology areas that "will clearly have a major impact across a wide range of industries within the next 3 to 5 years. "2 Gartner also listed parallel architectures and data mining as two of the top 10 new technologies in which companies will invest during the next 5 years. According to a recent Gartner HPC Research Note, "With the rapid advance in data capture, transmission and storage, large-systems users will increasingly need to implement new and innovative ways to mine the after-market value of their vast stores of detail data, employing MPP [massively parallel processing] systems to create new sources of business advantage (0.9 probability)." The most commonly used techniques in data mining are:

- **Artificial neural networks**: Non-linear predictive models that learn through training and resemble biological neural networks in structure.
- **Decision trees**: Tree-shaped structures that represent sets of decisions. These decisions generate rules for the classification of a dataset. Specific decision tree

methods include Classification and Regression Trees (CART) and Chi Square Automatic Interaction Detection (CHAID).

- **Genetic algorithms**: Optimization techniques that use process such as genetic combination, mutation, and natural selection in a design based on the concepts of evolution.
- **Nearest neighbor method**: A technique that classifies each record in a dataset based on a combination of the classes of the k record(s) most similar to it in a historical dataset (where k^3-1). Sometimes called the k-nearest neighbor technique.
- **Rule induction**: The extraction of useful if-then rules from data based on statistical significance.

Many of these technologies have been in use for more than a decade in specialized analysis tools that work with relatively small volumes of data. These capabilities are now evolving to integrate directly with industry-standard data warehouse and OLAP platforms. The appendix to this white paper provides a glossary of data mining terms.

1.7. DATA ANALYSIS

Analysis of data is a process of inspecting, cleansing, transforming, and modeling data with the goal of discovering useful information, suggesting conclusions, and supporting decision-making (Zohuri and Moghaddam, 2017). Data analysis has multiple facets and approaches, encompassing diverse techniques under a variety of names, in different business, science, and social science domains.

Data mining is a particular data analysis technique that focuses on modeling and knowledge discovery for predictive rather than purely descriptive purposes. Business intelligence covers data analysis that relies heavily on aggregation, focusing on business information. In statistical applications, some people divide data analysis into descriptive statistics, Exploratory Data Analysis (EDA), and Confirmatory Data Analysis (CDA) (Valverde-Albacete et al., 2016). EDA focuses on discovering new features in the data and CDA on confirming or falsifying existing hypotheses. Predictive analytics focuses on application of statistical models for predictive forecasting or classification, while text analytics applies statistical, linguistic, and structural techniques to extract and classify information from textual sources, a species of unstructured data. All are varieties of data analysis. There are two forms of data analysis that can be used for extracting models describing important classes or to predict future data trends. These two forms are as follows –

- Classification
- Prediction

1.7.1. Classification

Classification models predict categorical class labels; and prediction models predict continuous valued functions (Gorade et al., 2017). For example, we can build a classification model to categorize bank loan applications as either safe or risky, or a prediction model to predict the expenditures in dollars of potential customers on computer equipment given their income and occupation. Following are the examples of cases where the data analysis task is Classification –

- A bank loan officer wants to analyze the data in order to know which customers (loan applicant) are risky or which are safe.
- A marketing manager at a company needs to analyze a customer with a given profile, who will buy a new computer.

In both of the above examples, a model or classifier is constructed to predict the categorical labels. These labels are risky or safe for loan application data and yes or no for marketing data. With the help of the bank loan application that we have discussed above, let us understand the working of classification. The Data Classification process includes two steps -

- Building the Classifier or Model
- Using Classifier for Classification

Building the Classifier or Model

- This step is the learning step or the learning phase.
- In this step the classification algorithms build the classifier.

- The classifier is built from the training set made up of database tuples and their associated class labels.
- Each tuple that constitutes the training set is referred to as a category or class. These tuples can also be referred to as sample, object or data points.

The training phase of classification algorithm is shown in the following figure 1.4.

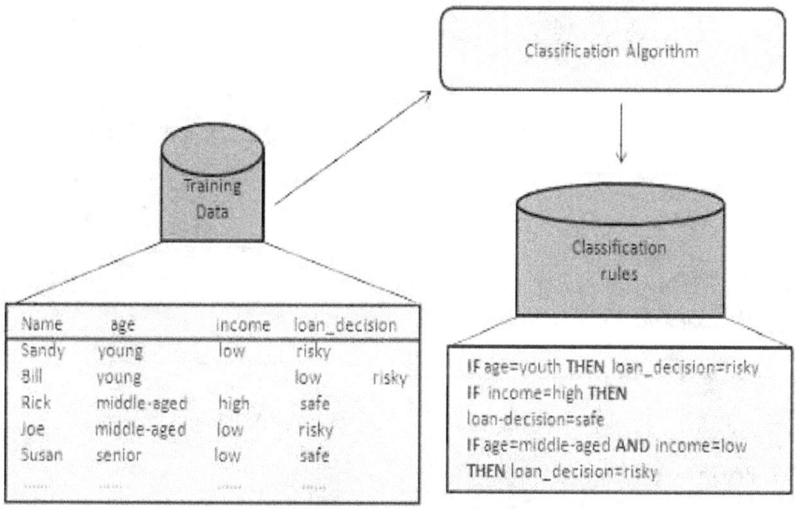

Figure 1.4. Training phase of classification algorithm

Using Classifier for Classification: In this step, the classifier is used for classification. Here the test data is used to estimate the accuracy of classification rules. The classification rules can be applied to the new data tuples if the accuracy is considered acceptable. The testing phase of classifier is shown in the following figure 1.5.

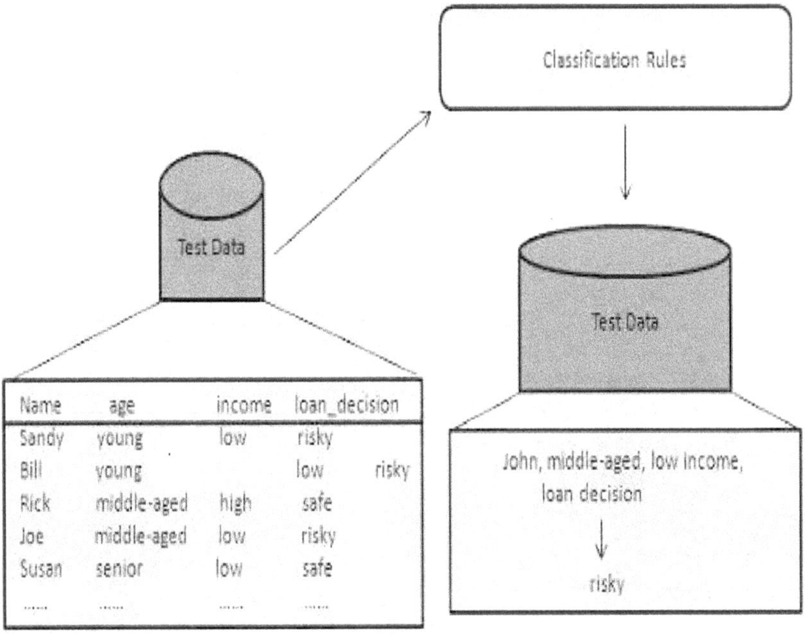

Figure 1.5. Testing phase of classification

1.7.2. Prediction

Following are the examples of cases where the data analysis task is Prediction - Suppose the marketing manager needs to predict how much a given customer will spend during a sale at his company.

In this example we are bothered to predict a numeric value. Therefore the data analysis task is an example of numeric prediction. In this case, a model or a predictor will be constructed that predicts a continuous-valued-function or ordered value. Regression analysis is a statistical methodology that is most often used for numeric prediction (Amirian et al., 2017).

1.7.3. Classification and Prediction Issues

The major issue is preparing the data for Classification and Prediction. Preparing the data involves the following activities –

- Data Cleaning – Data cleaning involves removing the noise and treatment of missing values. The noise is removed by applying smoothing techniques and the problem of missing values is solved by replacing a missing value with most commonly occurring value for that attribute.
- Relevance Analysis – Database may also have the irrelevant attributes. Correlation analysis is used to know whether any two given attributes are related.
- Data Transformation and reduction – The data can be transformed by any of the following methods.
    - Normalization – The data is transformed using normalization. Normalization involves scaling all values for given attribute in order to make them fall within a small specified range. Normalization is used when in the learning step, the neural networks or the methods involving measurements are used.
    - Generalization – The data can also be transformed by generalizing it to the higher concept. For this purpose we can use the concept hierarchies.

Data can also be reduced by some other methods such as wavelet transformation, binning, histogram analysis, and clustering. Here is the criterion for comparing the methods of Classification and Prediction

- Accuracy – Accuracy of classifier refers to the ability of classifier. It predicts the class label correctly and the accuracy of the predictor refers to how well a given predictor can guess the value of predicted attribute for a new data.
- Speed – this refers to the computational cost in generating and using the classifier or predictor.
- Robustness – It refers to the ability of classifier or predictor to make correct predictions from given noisy data.

- Scalability – Scalability refers to the ability to construct the classifier or predictor efficiently; given large amount of data.
- Interpretability – It refers to what extent the classifier or predictor understands.

1.8. FEATURE SELECTION FOR CLASSIFICATION

As the dimensionality of the data increases, many types of data analysis and classification problems become significantly harder (Santhanam et al., 2016). Sometimes the data also becomes increasingly sparse in the space it occupies. This can lead to big problems for both supervised and unsupervised learning. On the one hand, in the case of supervised learning or classification the available training data may be too small, i.e, there may be too few data objects to allow the creation of a reliable model for assigning a class to all possible objects. On the other hand, for unsupervised learning methods or clustering algorithms, various vitally important definitions like density or distance between points may become less convincing. As a result, a high number of features can lead to lower classification accuracy and clusters of poor quality. High dimensional data is also a serious problem for many classification algorithms due to its high computational cost and memory usage.

The size of the dataset can be measured in two dimensions and they are: number of features (N) and number of instances (P). In the present scenario, both N and P are enormously large. This leads to the fact that there is a need to identify the subset of features according to a certain criterion and this can be used as tool to study the datasets. When N (i.e. the number of features) is reduced, the value of P (i.e. the number of instances) gets automatically reduced, and the size of the overall dataset shrinks and a small unique dataset is formed which is devoid of unwanted, irrelevant and duplicate features and is ready for further analysis. Therefore, it can be stated that the basic motto of feature selection techniques is to find and learn some unique functions from the patterns available from the dataset undertaken for study and then makes the new pattern recognized by these learning functions.

Feature selection is the process of selecting a subset of the terms occurring in the training set and using only this subset as features in text classification. Feature selection serves two main purposes. First, it makes training and applying a classifier more efficient by decreasing the size of the effective vocabulary. This is of particular importance for classifiers that, unlike NB, are expensive to train. Second, feature selection often increases classification accuracy by eliminating noise features.

A noise feature is one that, when added to the document representation, increases the classification error on new data. Suppose a rare term, say arachnocentric, has no information about a class, say China, but all instances of arachnocentric happen to occur in China documents in our training set. Then the learning method might produce a classifier that mis-assigns test documents containing arachnocentric to China. Such an incorrect generalization from an accidental property of the training set is called over fitting.

From the perspective of machine learning it is realized that the existence of too many features (genes) may leads into over-fitting and also the reduction of classification performance. For example, if we build a classifier from the full set of features, a large number of classifiers may fit the training data but many of them will have weak prediction ability. This is because most of the features are not associated to the predicted parameter.

Therefore, the feature selection process plays a vital role for the construction of a successful classifier from the gene expression data. So, it is very important to identify the features that influence the prediction parameter and the prediction performance.

It is demonstrated that feature selection is an effective way of eliminating the redundant and irrelevant features thereby enhancing the efficiency in learning tasks, enhancing learning performance like predictive accuracy, enhancing comprehensibility of the outcome and reduction of the storage space. The general procedure for feature selection has four key steps as shown in figure 1.6.

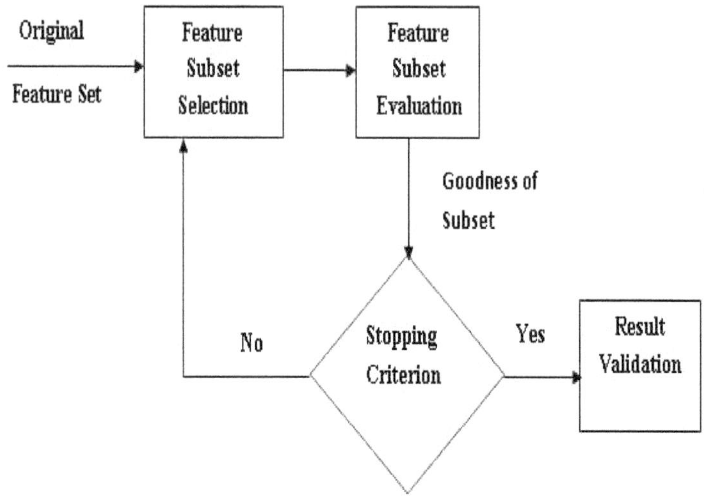

Figure 1.6. Steps in Feature Selection Process

- Feature Subset Selection
- Feature Subset Evaluation
- Stopping Criteria
- Result Validation

Feature Subset Selection is a heuristic search in which each state specifies a candidate subset for evaluation in the search space (Zarshenas and Suzuki, 2016). Two basic factors which influence the nature of the subset selection process are search starting point and search organization. The search starting point decides the direction of search. The available methods are going forward, moving backward, hybrid method, weighting, and random methods. The search organization is responsible for the feature selection process with a specific strategy, such as sequential search, exponential search or random search. In the next step the newly generated subset must be evaluated by a certain evaluation criteria. Many evaluation criteria have been proposed in the literature to analyze the effectiveness of the different subgroup of features that are generated. The evaluation criteria can be categorized into two groups: independent and dependent criteria.

Independent criteria exploit the essential characteristics of the training data without involving any mining algorithms to evaluate the goodness of a feature set or feature. The dependent criteria involve predetermined mining algorithms for feature selection. Among the generated feature subset the one that gives highest performance for mining algorithm will be selected. The process will be stopped when the stopping criteria is satisfied. Feature selection process ends with validation procedure. It is not the part of feature selection process but feature selection method must be validated by carrying out different tests and comparisons with previously established results or comparison with the results of competing methods by simulated datasets, real world datasets or both.

1.9. RESEARCH MOTIVATION

Medical diagnosis is treated to be an important yet delicate job, which has to be performed with precision and efficiency. Its automation would be greatly advantageous. Clinical decisions are frequently made based on the intuition and experience of the doctor more than based on the knowledge abundant data that stays concealed in the repository, that results in unnecessary biases, errors and huge medical expenses that impacts the quality of service given to patients. Data mining provides the means to create a knowledge-rich environment that can aid to take accurate clinical decisions.

1.10. PROBLEM SPECIFICATION

The use of data mining in the development of healthcare is seeing a manifold increase due to the rich information available with the health sector and data mining has emerged to be an indispensable process in the recent times. Lately, in the medicinal sector, several diseases are diagnosed with the help of evolutionary techniques and several research works have been carried out combined with rough set theories. Also, evolutionary technique is utilized for the prediction of heart disease, which is deemed the important reason behind health failure. Importantly, medical dataset are provided as an input to proposed system. These datasets are analyzed to find the heart disease occurrence. At last, it will provide an accurate decision so as to detect the heart disease.

1.11. OBJECTIVE OF THE RESEARCH

The main concern is to find the heart diseases since the number of deaths due to heart disease has alarmingly increased worldwide. The main goal of the research work is described as follows: "To study about the phases of heart diseases prediction by use of optimization techniques, To implement a technique that focus on risk factors, To propose an method that increases classification accuracy with reduced number of iterations for convergence, To compare and analyze the proposed systems with existing methods artificial neural network, Coronary Heart Disease prediction using Particle Swarm Optimization Approach and provide the best solution".

1.12. RESEARCH CONTRIBUTION

The major contributions of this research work are listed below:

- The first contribution is the development of Noise aware Optimal Risk Factor Selection for Heart Disease Prediction System (NORFS-HDPS),
- The second contribution is the development of Alpha Rough Set Theory combined with Fuzzy SVM (ARST-FSVM) Based Classification for Prediction
- The third contribution is the development of Hybrid Rough Set-Hybrid Multi Class SVM (HRS-HMCSVM) for the accurate prediction of heart disease"

1.13. OVERALL ORGANIZATION OF THE THESIS

The overall organization of the research method is given as follows: In this chapter 1, overview of heart disease and their risk factors has been discussed in detailed. And the role of data mining techniques and detailed description about the data mining has also been given.

In chapter 2, varying related research methodologies to predict and diagnosis the heart disease has been discussed. The different research methodologies are provided with the clear description of working procedure is given.

In chapter 3, Introducing novel research framework namely Noise aware Optimal Risk Factor Selection for Heart Disease Prediction System (NORFS-HDPS) is discussed in detail with required examples and explanation

In chapter 4, Alpha Rough Set Theory combined with Fuzzy SVM (ARST-FSVM) Based Classification for Prediction is discussed in detail with suitable examples and explanation

In chapter 5, Hybrid Rough Set-Hybrid Multi Class SVM (HRS-HMCSVM) for the accurate prediction of heart disease is introduced and discussed in detail with required examples and explanation. This system has been discussed in detail with suitable procedure and explanation.

In chapter 6, overall results and discussion of the proposed research methodologies has been discussed with percentage evaluation

Finally in chapter 7, final conclusion of the research methodologies based on results obtained were discussed in detail.

1.14. SUMMARY

In this chapter, discussion about the heart disease prediction and their symptoms has been discussed in detailed. And also discussion about the data mining techniques which can be used to diagnosis the heart disease has been discussed in detail. This chapter provides the short overview of the heart disease occurrence in depth.

1.15. OVERALL RESEARCH PROCESS DIAGRAM

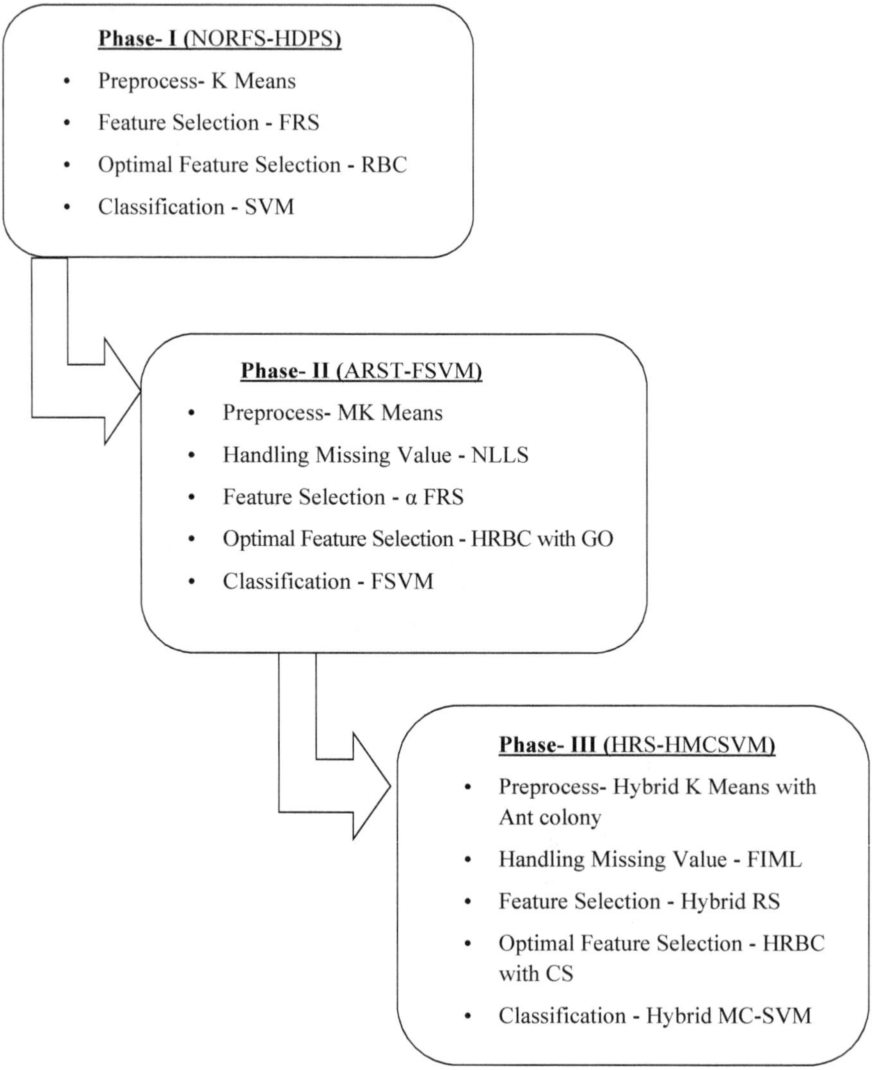

CHAPTER 2

LITERATURE SURVEY

2.1. INTRODUCTION

This chapter forms the motivation of this research work. In this chapter, the basis theories of heart disease data using data mining and big data, preprocessing, feature selection and classification methods will be reviewed. The chapter presents the literature of methods on preprocessing, optimization based feature selection methods and classification algorithms.

2.2. METHODS OF PREPROCESSING DATA

Mohd et al. (2013) discussed data pre-processing tasks involving data interpretation; data integration, noisy data, missing data, and data inconsistency are presented. The dataset prepared includes all the fields that are required for the research, pertaining to oral cancer diagnosis with demographics, social habit, clinical symptoms, and histological variables. After data normalization and transformation, the finding of the study prepared oral cancer dataset with 27 attributes as a part of study contribution. There are only one continuous and one numerical variable, which are case_id and age. The remaining variables are discrete or categorical variables.

Bai et al. (2006) introduced a straightforward and effective chromatographic data pre-processing method developing for utilization prior to chemometric analysis of large metabonomic dataset arising from high performance liquid chromatography. Nucleotides chromatographic fingerprinting in human urines is employed to validate the method. Performance for discrimination cancer samples from healthy urinary sample with principal component analysis is advanced by this method. The first and second principal components could discriminate the two groups by a straight line with precision rate of 75% for cancer samples and 92% for normal samples. Using unprocessed data only 50% cancer samples could be discriminated from healthy cluster. This method is proved to be an effective chromatographic data pre-processing procedure in metabonomics.

Yoshida et al. (2016) a simple and effective preprocessing method for melanoma classification by considering cytological properties of melanomas, in particular the alignment of the major axis of the tumor in the same direction. It evaluates the method with a set of 1,760 dermoscopic images (329 of melanomas and 1,431 of nevi) and a simple Convolutional Neural Network (CNN) classifier with five-fold cross validation. The tumor alignment method improves the classification performance by 5.8% in terms of the Area Under the ROC Curve (AUC). In addition, it proves to be 2.1% better in term of AUC when compared with the same configured CNN trained using images that are nine times larger. The results also show that considering the intrinsic features of the classification target is important even when the classifier has a capability to obtain effective features automatically through its learning process.

Ch'ng et al. (2014) presents a two level k-means segmentation technique for eczema skin lesion segmentation. Two class criteria are used for classifying the normal skin and eczema skin lesions using Mahalanobis distance. In order to further improve the segmentation performance normalized color spaces are used. The experiments include RGB and CIE lab color models; and their Color Space Normalized-I (CSN-I) versions. For pre-processing Frankle-McCann retinex and adaptive light compensation is used. The experimental results show that our proposed algorithm gives better results with normalized color spaces. It achieved a segmentation accuracy of 86.07% for RGB normalized I color space for the G channel with adaptive light compensation.

Chayes et al. (2017) used a semi-supervised algorithm for processing and classification of hyper spectral imagery. For initialization, it keeps 20% of the data intact, and use Principal Component Analysis (PCA) to discard voxels from noisier bands and pixels. Then, it uses either an Accelerated Proximal Gradient algorithm (APGL), or a modified APGL algorithm with a penalty term for distance between unpainted pixels and end members (APGL Hyp), on the initialized data cube to unpainted the missing data. APGL and APGL Hyp are distinguished by performance on datasets with full pixels removed or extreme noise. It can also classify the unpainted cube by assigning each pixel to its nearest end member via Euclidean distance. It demonstrates improved accuracy in classification over data-mining techniques like k-means, immixing techniques like Hierarchical Non-Negative Matrix Factorization, and graph-based methods like Non-Local Total Variation.

Dewan et al. (2017) investigates the problem of clustering trajectory data and propose a novel algorithm for clustering similar full and sub-trajectories together while modeling uncertainty in this data. It describes the necessary pre-processing techniques for clustering trajectory data, namely techniques to discretize raw location data using Possible World semantics to capture the inherent uncertainty in location data, and to segment full trajectories in to meaningful sub-trajectories. As a baseline, it extends the well known K-means algorithm to cluster trajectory data.

Bilalli et al. (2017) addressed that the problem by automating the pre-processing with the support of meta-learning. To this end, it analyzed a wide range of data pre-processing techniques and a set of classification algorithms. For each classification algorithm that we consider and a given dataset, we are able to automatically suggest the transformations that improve the quality of the results of the algorithm on the dataset. This approach will help non-expert users to more effectively identify the transformations appropriate to their applications, and hence to achieve improved results.

Al Shalabi et al. (2006) discussed about that data pre processing deals with data preparation and data transformation and seek to improve the overall process of data mining and at the same time make the process of knowledge discovery more efficient. Incomplete records or missing values produce a challenge to data mining process and can lead to wrong interpretation of knowledge. An instance is called incomplete if there exist at least one missing or unknown value for any attribute. An instance may contain several missing values. Before applying machine learning approach, it is essential either replace the missing values with some appropriate values or to remove the instance having missing values.

Wüthrich et al. (2016) present the non-Gaussian character of glint noise is demonstrated by exploratory data analysis. This non-Gaussian behaviour is characterized by outliers in the form of glint spikes. Since glint noise is processed by an angle-tracking Kalman filter, and since the latter is quite non robust, strategies is proposed to minimize the effect of these glint spikes. One of the strategies, which involve robust pre processing of the data, is pursued in detail. Finally, some results of a planar missile simulation are presented that clearly demonstrate the merits of the robust pre processing strategy.

Stefanowski and Wilk (2008) describes a new approach to selective pre-processing of imbalanced data which combines local over-sampling of the minority class with filtering difficult examples from majority classes. It discusses problems of constructing classifiers from imbalanced data. Re-sampling approaches that change the original class distribution are often used to improve performance of classifiers for the minority class.

Lee et al. (2006) developed a multi-step strategy for data preprocessing and afterwards feature selection. The preprocessing is composed of binning, baseline correction, and normalization. For the preprocessed data, it use a new feature subset selection method. This scheme is applied to the analysis of ovarian cancer dataset to predict early relapse in ovarian cancer. To validate the performance of the algorithm, experiments are performed in comparison with other feature selection and classification methods.

2.3. REVIEWS ON HEART DISEASE

Intelligent and Effective Heart Attack Prediction (IEHPS) (Patil and Kumaraswamy, 2009) presents methodology for the extraction of significant patterns from the heart disease warehouses for heart attack prediction. Initially, the data warehouse is preprocessed to make the mining process more efficient. The preprocessed data warehouse is then clustered using the K-means clustering algorithm. Frequent Itemset Mining (FIM) is performed using MAFIA (MAximal Frequent Itemset Algorithm) for the extraction of association rules from the clustered dataset. Weightage is then calculated and the patterns vital to heart attack prediction are selected according to the weightage. The neural network is trained with the selected patterns. Multi-layer Perceptron model is used with Back-propagation as the training algorithm. The significant patterns are extracted with the aid of the significance weightage greater than the pre-defined threshold.

Jabbar et al. (2011) proposed Association Rule mining based on the sequence number and clustering for heart attack prediction. The entire database is divided into partitions of equal size. The dataset with 14 attributes was used in that work and also each cluster is considered one at a time for calculating frequent item sets. This approach reduces main memory requirement. To predict the heart attack in an efficient way the patterns are extracted from the database with significant weight calculation. The frequent patterns having a value greater than a predefined threshold were chosen for the valuable prediction of heart attack. Three mining goals were defined based on data exploration and all those models could answer complex queries in predicting heart attack.

Shouman et al. (2012) proposed k means clustering with the decision tree method to predict the heart disease. In their work they suggested several centroid selection methods for k-means clustering to increase efficiency. The 13 input attributes were collected from Cleveland Clinic Foundation Heart disease data set. The sensitivity, specificity, and accuracy are calculated with different initial centroids selection methods and different numbers of clusters. For the random attribute and random row methods, ten runs were executed and the average and best for each method were calculated. When comparing integrating k-means clustering and decision tree with traditional decision tree applied previously on the same data set in diagnosing heart disease patients. In Addition, integrating k means clustering and decision tree could achieve higher accuracy than the paging algorithm in the diagnosis of heart disease patients. The accuracy achieved was 83.9% by the enabler method with two clusters.

Frequently the proximity with regard to some defined distance measure (Nouir et al., 2007) is known as Clustering. The clustering problem has been identified in numerous contexts and addressed being proven beneficial in many medical applications. Clustering the medical data into small with meaningful data can aid in the discovery of patterns by supporting the extraction of numerous appropriate features from each of the clusters thereby introducing structure into the data and aiding the application of conventional data mining techniques.

Jabbar et al. (2011) proposed enhanced K means clustering algorithm for predicting coronary heart disease. There are two strategies are used for enhancing K-means clustering algorithm. First the author proposed weighted ranking algorithm to overcome the problem of random selection of initial centroids. Second the attributes associated with weights concerned by the physicians are taken into account in both ranking and the K-means algorithm instead of assigning unit weight to all the attributes. The heart dataset was collected from UCI machine learning repository. Moreover 35 conditions are carried out to assign weights to attributes. From an experiment the author concluded that the proposed algorithm improves the consistency and quality of the final clusters. The unique clusters generates in turns of consistency.

Sumathi and Kirubakaran (2012) the heart attack symptoms are predicted using biomedical data mining techniques. The author used data classification which is based on supervised machine learning algorithms. For data classification the Tanagra tool is used. Using entropy based cross validations and partitioned techniques, the data is evaluated and the results are compared. The algorithms used in these techniques are K- nearest neighbors, K-means and Mean Clustering Algorithm (EMC) is the extension of the K-mean algorithm for clustering process which reduces the number of iterations. As a result the author analyzed that the mean clustering algorithm performs well when compared to other algorithms. To run the data the time taken is very fast and it gives the result of accuracy about 82.90%. Further this work will enhanced by applying unsupervised machine learning algorithm.

Cleaning and filtering of the data might be necessarily carried out with respect to the data and data mining algorithm employed so as to avoid the creation of deceptive or inappropriate rules or patterns (Sekar and Rao, 2012). The steps involved in the pre-processing of a dataset are the removal of duplicate records, normalizing the values used to represent information in the database, accounting for missing data points and removing unneeded data fields. To make data appropriate for the mining process it needs to be transformed. The raw data is changed into data sets with a few appropriate characteristics. Moreover it might be essential to combine the data so as to reduce the number of data sets besides minimizing the memory and processing resources required by the data mining algorithm. This leads to removal of duplicate records and supplying the missing values in the heart disease data warehouse.

In addition, it is also transformed to a new form which is appropriate for clustering (Münz et al., 2007). Most of the existing methods use a k means and fuzzy k means clustering methods to group similar Cleveland dataset which is studied in literature. These clustering method initial number of selection of k number to predict different risk levels becomes difficult and missing attributes is simply replaced by zero

,so it reduce the clustering accuracy or the prediction results of heart disease. To address limitations of existing approaches a new technique based on NMF-HC and missing attribute imputation is done based on the Multi-Cycle Expectation Conditional Maximization (MCECM) for heart disease prediction is proposed.

2.4. FEATURE SELECTION METHODS ON HEART DISEASE DATA

Bermingham et al. (2015) investigated the effect of five feature selection approaches on the performance of a mixed model (G-BLUP) and a Bayesian (Bayes C) prediction method. We predicted height, High Density Lipoprotein cholesterol (HDL) and Body Mass Index (BMI) within 2,186 Croatian and into 810 UK individuals using genome-wide SNP data. Using all SNP information Bayes C and G-BLUP had similar predictive performance across all traits within the Croatian data, and for the highly polygenic traits height and BMI when predicting into the UK data. Bayes C outperformed G-BLUP in the prediction of HDL, which is influenced by loci of moderate size, in the UK data. Supervised feature selection of a SNP subset in the G-BLUP framework provided a flexible, generalizable and computationally efficient alternative to Bayes C; but careful evaluation of predictive performance is required when supervised feature selection has been used.

Acharya et al. (2015) presented a novel integrated index for prediction of SCD with a high level of accuracy by using Electro Cardio Gram (ECG) signals. To achieve this, nonlinear features (Fractal Dimension (FD), Hurst's exponent (H), Detrended Fluctuation Analysis (DFA), Approximate Entropy (ApproxEnt), Sample Entropy (SampEnt), and Correlation Dimension (CD)) are first extracted from the second level Discrete Wavelet Transform (DWT) decomposed ECG signal. The extracted nonlinear features are ranked using *t*-value and then, a combination of highly ranked features are used in the formulation and employment of an integrated Sudden Cardiac Death Index (SCDI). This calculated novel SCDI can be used to accurately predict SCD (four minutes before the occurrence) by using just one numerical value four minutes before the SCD episode. Also, the nonlinear features are fed to the following classifiers: Decision Tree (DT), k-Nearest Neighbor (KNN), and Support Vector Machine (SVM).

Sun et al. (2014) predicts the transition points at which hypertension is brought into, as well as pushed out of, control. In a cohort of 1294 patients with hypertension enrolled in a chronic disease management program at the Vanderbilt University Medical Center, patients are modeled as an array of features derived from the clinical domain over time, which are distilled into a core set using an information gain criteria regarding their predictive performance. A model for transition point prediction was then computed using a random forest classifier.

Inbarani et al. (2014) introduced new supervised feature selection methods based on hybridization of Particle Swarm Optimization (PSO), PSO based Relative Reduct (PSO-RR) and PSO based Quick Reduct (PSO-QR) are presented for the diseases diagnosis. The experimental result on several standard medical datasets proves the efficiency of the proposed technique as well as enhancements over the existing feature selection techniques.

Turkeli et al. (2003) investigated the effect of feature extraction and feature selection on clustering of the expression data on two different data sets for ovarian cancer. One data set consisted of 2176 transcripts from 30 samples, nine from normal ovarian epithelial cells and 21 from cancerous ones. The other data set had 7129 transcripts coming from 27 tumor and four normal ovarian tissues. Hierarchical clustering algorithms employing complete-link, average-link and Ward's method were implemented for comparative evaluation. PCA is applied for feature extraction and resulted in 100% segregation. Feature selection is performed to identify the most distinguishing genes using CART/spl reg/ software. Selected features were able to cluster the data with 100% success. The results suggest that adoption of feature extraction and selection enhances the quality of clustering of gene expression data for ovarian cancer. Identification of distinguishing genes is a more complex problem that requires incorporating pathway knowledge with statistical and machine learning methods.

Plant et al. (2006) presents a 3-step feature selection framework combining the advantages of efficient filter and effective wrapper techniques. It demonstrates the performance of framework on two SELDI-TOF-MS data sets for identifying biomarker candidates in ovarian and prostate cancer

Medjahed et al. (2017) presents a complete cancer diagnostic process through kernel-based learning and feature selection. First, Support Vector Machines Recursive Feature Elimination (SVM-RFE) is used to pre filter the genes. Second, the SVM-RFE is enhanced by using Binary Dragon Fly (BDF), which is a recently developed meta heuristic that has never been benchmarked in the context of feature selection. The objective function is the average of classification accuracy rate generated by three kernel-based learning methods. It conducted a series of experiments on six microarray datasets. Experiment results demonstrate that this approach is efficient and provides a higher classification accuracy rate using a reduced number of genes.

Danala et al. (2017) aimed to investigate the role of applying quantitative image features computed from Computed Tomography (CT) images for early prediction of tumor response to chemotherapy in the clinical trials for treating ovarian cancer patients. Two initial feature pools were built using image features computed from pre-therapy CT images only and image feature difference computed from both pre- and post-therapy images. A feature selection method was applied to select optimal features, and an equal-weighted fusion method was used to generate a new quantitative imaging marker from each pool to predict 6-month progression-free survival. The prediction accuracy between quantitative imaging markers and the Response Evaluation Criteria in Solid Tumors (RECIST) criteria was also compared.

Motieghader et al. (2017) used a hybrid meta-heuristic algorithm, which is an integration of Genetic Algorithm and Learning Automata (GALA). The time complexity of GALA is O(G.m.n3) and it has acceptable accuracy and performance on some well-known cancer datasets. To evaluate the performance of GALA, six different cancer datasets including Colon, ALL_AML, SRBCT, MLL, Tumors_9 and Tumors_11 are selected. Based on the evaluation process, the GALA algorithm provided remarkable results on each dataset compared to some recently used algorithms.

Wu et al. (2012) analyzes the performance of improvement GSO, a number of experiments are carried out on a set of well-known benchmark global optimization problems. The effects of the parameters about the improvement algorithms are discussed by uniform design experiment. Numerical results reveal that the algorithms can find better solutions when compared to classical GSO and other heuristic algorithms and are powerful search algorithms for various global optimization problems.

Dastider et al. (2015) used a binary particle swarm optimization (PSO) algorithm for feature selection in clustering. We aim at (i) Maximizing the Laplacian Score and (ii) Minimizing the inter-attribute correlation, and unifying the value using no preference method. Empirical studies have been conducted over 21 publicly available datasets. The average reduction is feature set cardinality is more than 71%. In terms of cluster validity also there is an efficiency of above 90%.

Zawbaa et al. (2015) used feature selection based on Social Spider Optimization (SSO). SSO is used in the system as searching method to find optimal feature set maximizing classification performance and mimics the cooperative behavior mechanism of social spiders in nature. The SSO algorithm considers two different search agents (social members) male and female spiders, that simulate a group of spiders with interaction to each other based on the biological laws of the cooperative colony. Depending on spider gender, each spider (individual) is simulating a set of different evolutionary operators of different cooperative behaviors that are typically found in the colony. This system is evaluated using different evaluation criteria on 18 different datasets, which compared with two common search methods namely particle swarm optimization (PSO), and Genetic Algorithm (GA). SSO algorithm proves an advance in classification performance using different evaluation indicators.

Liu et al. (2015) discussed multilevel threshold for color image segmentation using Cooperative Bacterial Foraging Algorithm (CBFA), which combined bacterial chemo taxis, cell-to-cell communication, and an adaptive foraging mechanism to extend original bacterial foraging algorithm. The superiority of the algorithm can reach a higher quality adequate segmentation and reduce the CPU processing time, which is demonstrated by comparing with other algorithm.

Nalluri et al. (2017) suggested Artificial Fish Swarm Optimization (AFSO) meta heuristic algorithm which is inspired by the fish behavior under water. The wrapper approach of AFSO with support vector machine (SVM) is used for finding the feature subset with a minimum number of features. This approach is tested on nine different datasets having binary and multiple imbalanced classes and correlated with other meta heuristic algorithms. The results show that the approach is providing high classification accuracy with features subset having fewer features.

Alipoor et al. (2010) developed a novel combinational feature selection method on high throughput SELDI-TOF mass-spectroscopy data for ovarian cancer classification. This method includes 3 steps: dataset normalization, dimensionality reduction using feature filtering, selecting the most informative features utilizing binary particle swarm optimization. Indeed, the method employs a combination of filter and wrapper feature selection methods to find features with high discriminatory power. The algorithm is successfully validated using a well-known ovarian cancer proteomic dataset. Results of applying the method are superior to state of the art methods in proteomic pattern recognition. It reduces extremely high dimensionality of proteomic data to 3 dimensional and linearly separable data. Therefore, this system clearly outperforms previous works in both respects of accuracy and number of required features; witch may lead in high accuracy and high speed diagnosis procedure.

Meng (2006) discussed a swarming-agent based intelligence algorithm using a hybrid Ant Colony Optimization/Particle Swarm Optimization (ACO/PSO) algorithm to identify the diagnostic proteomic patterns of biomarkers for early detection of ovarian cancer. The experimental results demonstrated that this system has high predictive accuracy and better diagnostic performance.

Jiang et al. (2010) used a novel liver cancer identification method based on PSO-SVM. First, the Region of Interest (ROI) is determined by Lazy-Snapping, and various texture features are extracted from ROI. Afterwards, F-score algorithm is applied to select relevant features, based on which liver cancer classifier is designed by combining parallel Support Vector Machine (SVM) with Particle Swarm Optimization (PSO) algorithm. PSO is used to automatically choose parameters for SVM, and the advantage is that it makes the choice of parameter more objective and avoids the conscious decision and subjectivity in the traditional SVM whose parameters are decided through trial and error. The experiment results on real-world datasets show that the proposed parallel PSO-SVM training algorithm improves the prediction accuracy of liver cancer.

Xue et al. (2013) discussed classification problems that often have a large number of features in the data sets, but not all of them are useful for classification. Irrelevant and redundant features may even reduce the performance. Feature selection aims to choose a small number of relevant features to achieve similar or even better classification performance than using all features. It has two main conflicting objectives of maximizing the classification performance and minimizing the number of features. This research presents multi-objective particle swarm optimization (PSO) for feature selection. The task is to generate a Pareto front of non dominated solutions (feature subsets). Then investigate two PSO-based multi-objective feature selection algorithms. The first algorithm introduces the idea of non dominated sorting into PSO to address feature selection problems. The second algorithm applies the ideas of crowding, mutation, and dominance to PSO to search for the Pareto front solutions. The two multi-objective algorithms are evaluated on 12 benchmark data sets.

Han (2010) have introduced a feature selection based on genetic algorithm for classification of pre-miRNAs. The information gain of feature and the redundancy among features are considered in this algorithm. It uses a filter method that is based on information gain and similarity. This feature selection would aim to select the features with more information gain for classification. At the same time, it avoids the redundant features where the value of similarity is greater.

Yu and Liu (2003) have used feature selection technique for high-dimensional data using a Fast Correlation-Based Filter solution (FCBF). In this work, they have introduced a novel concept for predominant correlation and proposed a fast filter method which can identify relevant features as well as redundancy among relevant features without pair wise correlation analysis. The efficiency and effectiveness of this method is demonstrated through extensive comparisons with other methods using real-world data of high dimensionality.

Li and Yin (2013) presented a multi-objective biogeography based optimization method to select the small subset of informative gene relevant to the classification. In this algorithm, firstly, the Fisher-Markov selector is used to choose the 60 top gene expression data. Secondly, to make biogeography based optimization suitable for the discrete problem,

Binary Biogeography Based Optimization, as called BBBO, is proposed based on a binary migration model and a binary mutation model. Then, Multi-Objective Binary Biogeography Based Optimization, as we called MOBBBO, is proposed by integrating the non-dominated sorting method and the crowding distance method into the BBBO framework. Finally, the MOBBBO method is used for gene selection, and support vector machine is used as the classifier with the Leave-One-Out Cross-Validation method (LOOCV). In order to show the effective and efficiency of the algorithm, it is tested on ten gene expression dataset benchmarks. Experimental results demonstrate that the proposed method is better or at least comparable with previous particle swarm optimization (PSO) algorithm and support vector machine (SVM).

2.5. CLASSIFICATION ALGORITHMS OF HEART DISEASE DATASET

Taneja (2013) in the year 2013 used data mining tool WEKA 3.6.4 in heart disease prediction system using J48 technique achieved 95.56% accuracy and using Naïve Bayes technique achieved 92.42% and using Neural Network achieved 94.85%. In this paper, various data mining techniques have been studied for the diagnosis of heart disease. The data for the study collected from PGI, Chandigarh which has a total of 15 attributes. A total of 7339 instances were trained. Of the 15, only 8 attributes were selected.

Subbalakshmi et al. (2011) in the year 2011 has developed a Decision Support in Heart disease Prediction System (DSHDPS) using Naïve Bayes data mining modeling technique to discover the relationship between variables in database in the healthcare industry. This model could answer the complex queries. It is resulted out as the most effective model in the prediction of heart disease.

Jabbar et al. (2013) in the year 2012 proposed evolutionary algorithm for heart disease prediction. They used the genetic algorithm to predict the heart diseases in Andhra Pradesh population. They used the Association Rule Mining based on the sequence number and clustering for heart attack prediction.

Feshki et al. (2016) proposed the improving the heart disease diagnosis by evolutionary algorithm of PSO and feed forward neural network. In this research the work has been provided on a particular dataset using classification and feature selection approach. And provide the best accurate criteria for heart dieses diagnosis. The assessment of selected features of classified methods also showed that PSO method along with Neural Networks of Feed Forward Back-Propagation has the best accurate criteria.

Kaur and Singh (2014) proposed review on heart disease prediction system using data mining techniques. Data mining provides the methodology and technology to transform mounds of data into useful information for decision making and use this data for the prediction of heart disease with good accuracy. So that the prediction by using data mining algorithm given efficient results. Applying data mining techniques to heart disease treatment data can provide as reliable performance as that achieved in diagnosing heart disease.

Soni et al. (2011) proposed predictive data mining for medical diagnosis. The problem of constraining and summarizing different algorithms of data mining used in the field of medical prediction are discussed. The focus is on using different algorithms and combinations of several target attributes for intelligent and effective heart attack prediction using data mining. They conclude that the accuracy of the Decision Tree and Bayesian Classification further improves after applying genetic algorithm to reduce the actual data size to get the optimal subset of attribute sufficient for heart disease prediction.

Lakshmi and Reddy (2015) proposed fast rule-based heart disease prediction using associative classification mining. This research uses associative classification which builds a classifier with prediction rules of high interestingness values using Associative Classification and rewarding approach and experimental results show that this work helps doctors in their diagnosis decisions.

Support Vector Machine (SVM) is a most popularly used supervised machine learning algorithm for both regression and classification challenges (Suthaharan, 2016). It performs classification by finding the hyper-plane that differentiates the two classes very well. Support Vectors are simply the co-ordinates of individual observation. Support Vector Machine is a frontier which best segregates the two classes by hyper-plane. The SVM classifier objective is to maximize the margin. In the below shown figure,

H1 does not separate the classes. H2 does, but only with a small margin. H3 separates them with the maximum margin. The margin is the distance between separating hyper-plane and the training samples that are closest to this hyper-plane.

Renz et al. (2002) examines the use of standardized blood-test data for classification of benign cysts and malignant conditions. It uses Multi-Layer Perceptron (MLP) networks for classification and show that it is even possible to distinguish between early and late stage cancers with an accuracy of up to 92.9 %. Furthermore, it deals with missing data, an inevitable problem in clinical research that is not yet well explored in the context of neural networks. It compares several intuitive heuristics to estimate missing data and show that MLP networks are a suitable tool to deal with incomplete inputs.

Misganaw and Vidyasagar (2015) point out the importance of making use of the order information when it is inherent to the problem. It demonstrates that algorithms that use this additional information outperform the algorithms that do not, on a case study of assigning one of four labels to the ovarian cancer patients on the basis of their time of progression-free survival. As an aside, it is also pointed out that the algorithms that make use of ordering information require fewer data normalizations. This aspect is important in biological applications, where data are plagued by variations in platforms and protocols, batch effects, and so on.

Karemore et al. (2010) comparison of PCA and fuzzy clustering techniques in classifying protein profiles (chromatogram) of homogenates of different tissue origins: Ovarian, Cervix, Oral cancers, which were acquired using HPLC-LIF (High Performance Liquid Chromatography-Laser Induced Fluorescence) method developed in our laboratory. Study includes 11 chromatogram spectra each from oral, cervical, ovarian cancers as well as healthy volunteers. Generally multivariate analysis like PCA demands clear data that is devoid of day-to-day variation, artifacts due to experimental strategies, inherent uncertainty in pumping procedure which is very common activities during HPLC-LIF experiment. Under these circumstances we demonstrate how fuzzy clustering algorithm like Gath Geva followed by Sammon mapping outperform PCA mapping in classifying various cancers from healthy spectra with classification rate up to 95 % from

60%. Methods are validated using various clustering indexes and shows promising improvement in developing optical pathology like HPLC-LIF for early detection of various cancers in all uncertain conditions with high sensitivity and specificity.

Jeng et al. (2005) studies an intelligent system, including a Support Vector Regression (SVR) and a similar analysis, for the classification of the ovarian cancer with microarray data. That is, steps in the classification include a feature selection step and a distance measure step. Firstly, the SVR is used to do the feature selection. That is, the SVR is applied to obtain the important genes of ovarian cancer for all samples of microarray data. At the same time, we can compute the frequency of the gene selection based on the results of SVR for all samples to determine the target genes of ovarian cancer. Secondly, the distance under the similar analysis between target data and test data can be determined. From the distance results, the classification of ovarian cancer can easy to determine

Razak et al. (2016) discussed to circumvent these problems in data analysis stage with a machine learning technique called Random Forest. This system achieved 93.48 % accuracy for gastric cancer and 100 % accuracy for ovarian cancer. The results are promising and encouraging. Despite much noise contaminated the sample preparation process and low miRNA count in body fluids, this system able to identify miRNA markers responsible for classification of cancer.

Kumar and Rama Krishnan (2014) presents the usage of Extreme Learning Machines for cancer microarray gene expression data. Extreme Learning Machines overcomes the problems of over fitting, local minima and improper training rate that are most common in traditional algorithms. We have evaluated the binary classification performance of Extreme Learning Machines on five bench marked datasets of cancer microarray gene expression data namely ALL/AML, CNS, Lung Cancer, Ovarian Cancer and Prostate Cancer. Feature extraction has been performed using correlation coefficient prior to classification. The results indicate that ELM produces comparable or better results compared to the traditional classification methods like naive bayes, bagging, random forest and decision table.

Khazendar et al. (2014) used new method for automatic ovarian tumor classification based on decision level fusion. This method first extracts two different types of features (Histogram and Local Binary Pattern) from ultrasound images of the ovary. Support Vector Machine (SVM) is then used to classify ovarian tumor based on each type of features separately. The method then employs a novel decision fusion that categorizes SVM-based decision scores into a measure of confidence to assist the final diagnostic decision making. Experimental results on 187 ultrasound images of ovarian tumor show classification accuracy of 90%, 81% and 69% based on classification decisions of high, medium and low confidence respectively, whereas 18% of the cases were unclassified as inconclusive not sure cases. The paper argues that such confidence based prediction outcomes are more meaningful than other classical alternatives and closer to the reality in diagnosis of ovarian cancers.

Park et al. (2014) develop multi category classification models with optimal parameters and features; it systematically evaluated three machine learning algorithms and three feature selection methods using five-fold cross validation and a grid search. The study included 22 subjects with normal ovarian surface epithelial cells, 12 with SBOTs, and 79 with SOCs according to microarray data with 54,675 probe sets obtained from the national center for biotechnology information gene expression omnibus repository. Application of the optimal model of support vector machines one-versus-rest with signal-to-noise as a feature selection method gave an accuracy of 97.3%, relative classifier information of 0.916, and a kappa index of 0.941. In addition, 5 features, including the expression of putative biomarkers SNTN and AOX1, are selected to differentiate between normal, SBOT, and SOC groups. An accurate diagnosis of ovarian tumor subclasses by application of multi category machine learning would be cost-effective and simple to perform, and would ensure more effective subclass-targeted therapy.

Kim (2009) presents a novel method based on spectral bi-partitioning, traditionally used for finding min-cuts in graphs, for classification of cancer using microarray data. This method is applied to five publicly available datasets of acute leukemia, colon cancer, ovarian cancer, prostate cancer and diffuses large B-cell lymphoma, and is shown to have classification accuracy comparable to that of some of the currently known best classification methods for microarray data.

Chen et al. (2009) used supervised SVD approach to extract the gene features linked to chemotherapy response patients of ovarian cancer, and applied across factor normalization to remove the influences of the factors. Chi square test is used to detect whether the factors affect the distribution of chemotherapy response and quantile-quantile plot is used to detect the distribution of chemotherapy response samples. The experimental results show that the influences of the factors are removed effectively, and the classification performance of gene markers selected by the methods outperform that by SVMRFE and T-test in seven classifiers except for JRip classifier and Naïve Bayes classifier.

Knapp et al. (2017) discussed bioactive sphingo lipids play an essential role in the development and progression of cancer and they also take part in the process of metastasizing. This study suggests that some sphingo lipids can be used as potential biomarkers of advanced ovarian cancer and that they can play an important role in the pathogenesis of this disease.

Tseng et al. (2017) used ensemble learning and five data mining approaches, including support vector machine (SVM), C5.0, Extreme Learning Machine (ELM), Multivariate Adaptive Regression Splines (MARS), and Random Forest (RF), are integrated to rank the importance of risk factors and diagnose the recurrence of ovarian cancer. The medical records and pathologic status were extracted from the Chung Shan Medical University Hospital Tumor Registry. Experimental results illustrated that the integrated C5.0 model is a superior approach in predicting the recurrence of ovarian cancer. Moreover, the classification accuracies of C5.0, ELM, MARS, RF, and SVM indeed increased after using the selected important risk factors as predictors. Our findings suggest that The International Federation of Gynecology and Obstetrics (FIGO), Pathologic M, Age, and Pathologic T were the four most critical risk factors for ovarian cancer recurrence.

Maruf and Rashid (2011) used novel technique for dimensionality reduction of the SELDI-TOF data using wavelet decomposition. This technique is self adaptive and independent of the properties of data set. For classification purpose SVM has been introduced. The performance of the algorithm is evaluated on ovarian and pancreatic cancer data set. The data sets are collected from National Cancer Institute, Center for Cancer Research, USA. A comparative performance analysis with another recently reported algorithm in literature reveals that our method can reduce the dimensionality of the data set more effectively with improved classification accuracy, sensitivity and specificity.

Vance et al. (2010) used the high dimensional spectroscopy data is preprocessed using linear dimensionality reduction technique of principal component analysis and then classification is performed using support vector machines (SVM) and Adaptive Local Hyper plane (ALH). The influence of the number of extracted features as well as the parameters of the classification algorithms to the classification accuracy is also investigated. The experiments performed on real life data suggest that both classification methods are quite efficient in distinguishing among four types of proteins and they have a fairly robust detection performance for a range of the numbers of extracted features as well as the algorithms' parameters.

Sehgal et al. (2004) investigates the performance of different classification, Missing Value Estimation (MVE) and data dimension reduction techniques for the classification of gene expression data for BRCA1, BRCA2 and Sporadic mutations of epithelial ovarian cancer. Bayesian MVE and zero imputation techniques were employed to deal with missing values. This study showed the better performance of the Bayesian technique. A novel approach is introduced to use Generalized Regression Neural Network (GRNN) as genetic mutation classifier which completely outperformed both well established support vector machine and probabilistic neural network.

Maurya et al. (2014) discussed an automated system for detection and classification of one of the skin four types of skin cancers: Melanoma, Basal cell carcinoma, actinic Keratosis, Squamous cell carcinoma. There are a certain features of these types of skin cancers, which can be extracted using proper feature extraction algorithm. The features of skin lesions are extracted normalized symmetrical Grey Level Co-occurrence Matrices (GLCM). GLCM based texture features are extracted from each of the four classes and given as input to the Multi-Class Support vector machine which is used for c1assification purpose. It c1assifies the given data set into one of the four skin cancer classes. The accuracy of our proposed method is 81.43%.

Tan et al. (2005) utilized Fuzzy Neural Network (FNN) approach for assisting the diagnosis and analysis process. Amongst FNN, complementary learning FNN is able to rapidly derive fuzzy sets and formulate fuzzy rules. Complementary learning FNN uses positive and negative learning, and hence it sub sides the effect of curse of dimension and is capable of modeling the dynamics of problem space with relative good classification performance. Furthermore, FALCON-AART has human-like reasoning that allows physician to examine its computation in a familiar way. FALCON-AART can generate intuitive fuzzy rule to justify its reasoning, which is important to generate trust among the users of the system. Hence, FALCON-AART is applied in ovarian cancer diagnosis as a clinical decision support system in this work. Its experimental results are encouraging.

Mukhopadhyay et al. (2009) presented a technique for cancer classification based on multi objective genetic fuzzy clustering. The coordinates of the cluster centers have been fixed in the chromosomes and three fuzzy cluster strength indices are concurrently optimized. The resultant Pareto-optimal set solutions can be made better by a technique based on SVM classification. The final step involves clustering the non-dominated solutions information and combining them using a voting ensemble approach to yield clustering result. The performance of the multi objective clustering method has been compared with other algorithms with the available benchmark cancer data.

Saravanan and Rangasamy (2009) focused to develop classification algorithms for cancer gene expression with minimum gene subsets. Gene ranking can be performed with classical statistical techniques and two classifiers are used for gene selection and prediction. The result proves that support vector machine one-against-all (SVM-OAA) is superior to Linear Discriminator Analysis (LDA). It focused on accuracy with minimum gene subset and to predict the type of cancer.

Osareh and Shadgar (2010) carried out a micro array data analysis for the classification of cancer. A computerized system is formed for producing a reliable cancer analysis based on gene microarray expression data. Micro array data sets are selected which contains both binary and multi-class cancer problems. Many classifiers such as K-Nearest Neighbors, naive Bayes, Neural Networks, decision tree and SVM are used for classification. In particular, various experiments were carried out and their results are compared. From this result, the better classification model is predicted by the use of SVM classifier.

Sheng et al. (2009) used a Block Diagonal Linear Discriminator Analysis (BDLDA) which is improved and applied onto gene expression data. BDLDA is a classification tool along with embedded feature selection which has showed good performance on modeled data. But again, by employing cross validation in training, BDLDA involves lot of time consumption, therefore not a suitable algorithm for gene expression data that has a huge number of features and considerably small number of samples. In our algorithm, estimated error rate acts as a measure to select the best model. The algorithm is optimized by the repetition of the model construction procedure with earlier selected features eliminated, thus leading to a high classification robustness.

2.6. SUMMARY

This chapter explains about different literatures of the heart disease prediction methods, preprocessing, optimization based feature selection algorithms, classification methods and the relevant concepts for the efficient design of the proposed research. This chapter points out the advantages and disadvantages in the already available research works forming the core of the models proposed.

CHAPTER 3

OPTIMAL RISK FACTOR SELECTION APPROACH TO PREDICT HEART DISEASE

Heart disease becomes the most found disease in the world over people with all age. There is various research methods has been introduced earlier for the accurate prediction of heart disease. In the existing research method heart disease prediction is done by using Particle Swarm Optimization (PSO) algorithm which selects risk factors selection and the disease prediction is done by using decision tree method. However this method degrades in its performance with reduced accuracy due to more computational complexity of the PSO and decision tree algorithms. This method reduced in its performance in case of presence of more noises and less information present in the dataset. These problems are resolved in the proposed research methodology by introducing novel research framework namely Noise aware Optimal Risk Factor Selection for Heart Disease Prediction System (NORFS-HDPS). In this work, initially Pre-processing is done by using K-means clustering Algorithm to make the dataset cleaner, consistent and noise free. Then Feature reduction of the dataset is done by using Fuzzy based rough set theory. The fuzzy rough sets extend the rough set concept through the use of fuzzy equivalence classes. From this reduced feature set, optimal feature selection is done by using Improved Bee Colony approach. Finally, classification of dataset is done by using Support vector machine.

3.1. INTRODUCTION

Heart disease is the most common found disease in the real world environment which might cause various effects on the human health level (Rajeswari et al., 2012). Heart disease presence on humans might cause sudden death which requires to be identified as soon as possible for the prevention. More importantly older peoples frequently affected by heart disease and hospitalized which requires to be identified as soon as possible for the accurate and early identification of the heart disease (Shilaskar, and Ghatol 2013). Finding the heart disease early is most difficult task which requires knowledge on heart disease parameters. It is required to focus on the varying heart disease parameter values which varies based on varying age people health levels (Zhang et al., 2014).

However the optimal management and handling of heart disease factors gathered from multiple patients who are hospitalized in nature would be more difficult task (Schmidt et al., 2015). In this proposed research method, optimal handling of heart disease prediction is focused in order to deviate the heart disease prediction outcomes (Shah et al., 2017). The proposed research method attempts to focus on the varying heart disease characteristics and personal details about the patients to differentiate the effects of heart disease occurring on patients (Rao et al., 2013). There is various research methods has been proposed earlier which attempts to focus on accurate and reliable prediction of heart disease (Karystianis et al., 2015). However those techniques cannot predict accurately due to presence of varying risk factors such as pollution effects, varying noises present in the environment and so on. And also available research method are more cost in nature which cannot response well on time, thus the earlier prediction of heart disease would be more difficult task (Matsunaga et al., 2017).

In the proposed research methodology, accurate and early prediction of heart disease system is implemented which attempts to predict the occurrence of heart disease earlier based on risk factors that reflects the heart disease presents on humans. This study focuses on various samples that are gathered from the multiple patients for the accurate prediction of heart disease. From those samples, heart disease prediction is done based on the various risk factors such as pulse rate, blood pressure level and so on. This is ensured by introducing novel research framework namely Noise aware Optimal Risk Factor Selection for Heart Disease Prediction System (NORFS-HDPS)

3.2. OVERVIEW OF HEART DISEASE PREDICTION SYSTEM

Data mining is the process of analyzing data from different perspectives and summarizing it into useful information. It is an iterative and interactive process of discovering novel, valid, useful, comprehensive and understandable patterns and models in MASSIVE data sources. Data mining brings a set of tools and techniques that can be applied to processed medical data to discover hidden patterns that provide healthcare professionals an additional source of knowledge for making decisions. Medical data mining is Applying data mining techniques and methods in medical data. The challenge faced by healthcare industry with regard to the massive data-rich but information-poor collection is to extract valuable information to be available at a particular time, place in the form needed to support the decision-making process.

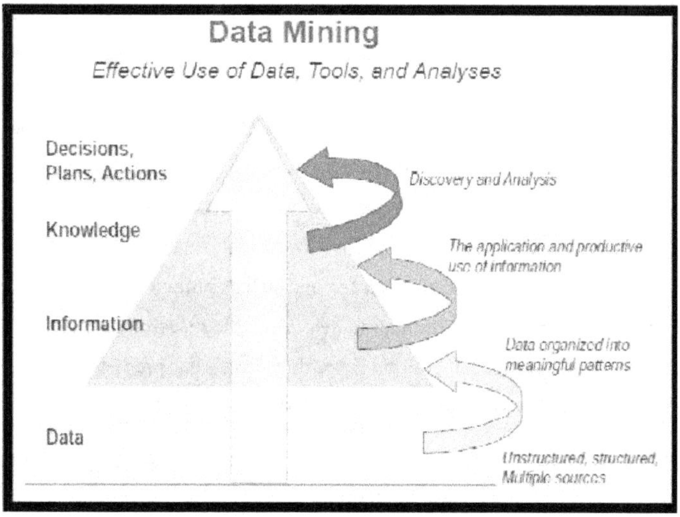

Figure 3.1. Transformation of data into decisions

Data mining consists of five major tasks:

- Extract, transform, and load transaction data onto the data warehouse system.
- Store and analyze the data in a multidimensional database system
- Provide data access to business analysts and information technology professionals
- Present the data in a useful format, such as a graph or table

3.2.1. Heart Disease

A heart attack occurs when one or more coronary arteries that supply blood to your heart muscle become blocked off. Medically, it is referred to as a myocardial infarction or MI. If the blood supply is cut off for more than a certain period of time, usually about 20 minutes, the muscle cells in the heart which are supplied by that artery may die. Human heart structure is shown in the following figure 3.2.

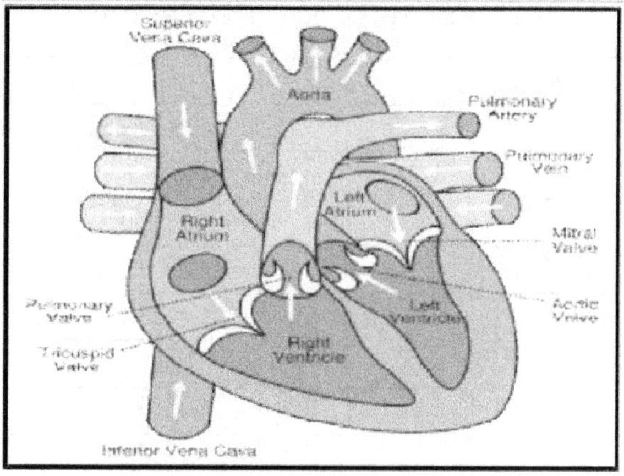

Figure 3.2. Human Heart Structure

3.2.2. Medical Data Mining

Applying data mining techniques in medical data to extract meaningful patterns and knowledge is called "Medical Data mining". With the widespread use of databases and explosive growth in their sizes, the healthcare industry faced with the problem of information overloading. Data mining provides the methodology and technology to transform these mounds of data into useful information for decision making.

3.2.3. Heart Disease Prediction System

Heart Disease Prediction System aims to exploit the various data mining techniques on medical data set to assist in the prediction of the heart disease. Many data mining techniques like classification, clustering, regression and artificial neural networks can be used for heart disease prediction. Following are the 14 main attributes widely used for the prediction of heart disease.

Table 3.1: Important attributes used for heart disease prediction

Attributes	Range
Age	Children, adults and not adults
Gender	Male / Female
Blood pressure	100/70 to 150/90
Cholesterol(LDL)	100 to 189
Heredity	40%
Blood sugar	80-120
PQ value	21.6-76
ST value	9.89-27.63
QT value	22.022-154
QRS value	8.532-68
R value	104-324
Heart beat rate	70-100
BMI	Men < 27 and Women < 25
Smoking habit	Yes/No
Alcohol intake	Yes/No
Mental stress	Yes/No

3.3. RISK FACTORS AWARE HEART DISEASE PREDICTION SYSTEM

In the proposed research method, early heart disease prediction system is focused which attempts to retrieve the heart disease risk factors in the accurate way. This is done with the concern of risk factors of heart disease which reflects the heart disease presence in the accurate way. This is ensured in the proposed research method by introducing the Noise aware Optimal Risk Factor Selection for Heart Disease Prediction System (NORFS-HDPS). This research work can ensure the optimal prediction of heart disease presence earlier, thus the proper treatment can be carried out on right time. However the information gathered from online regarding heart disease would consist of various noises and irrelevant information which would cause the accurate detection rate of heart disease.

This can be avoided by removing the noisy data and making them in the structured format, thus the accurate heart disease prediction can be ensured. The steps followed in the proposed research methodologies are given as follows:

- Preprocessing using K-means clustering Algorithm to make the dataset cleaner, consistent and noise free.
- Feature Selection of the dataset using Fuzzy based Rough set theory. The fuzzy rough sets extend the rough set concept through the use of fuzzy equivalence classes.
- Optimal feature selection using Improved Bee Colony approach
- Classification using Support vector machine is used for classification of the dataset

The overall flow of the proposed research method is given in figure 3.3.

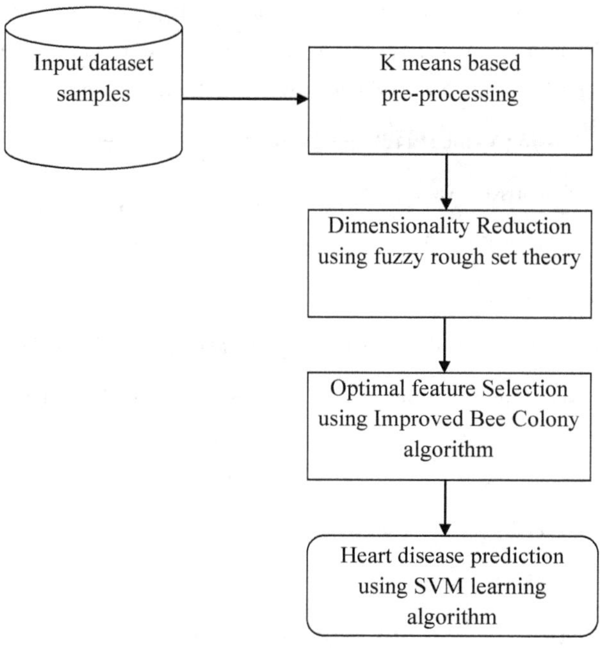

Figure 3.3. Overall proposed research work flow

3.3.1. Preprocessing Using K-Means Algorithm

Missing data values plays a more important role in the prediction process, where the incomplete information would lead to wrong prediction result of heart disease prediction. Incomplete information would lead to wrong prediction outcome which might cause the treatments, thus the dangerous effects patients might occur. In the proposed research method, missing value handling is done by using the K means algorithm.

K means algorithm is a most popular clustering technique from the data mining field whose main goal is to group the similar kind of data that are having same characteristics together. Here similarity is identified by using the Euclidean distance which can find the similarity between the multiple objects. Thus the grouping can be done more effectively. This distance similarity metric can be utilized to replace the missing values present in the database, thus the complete information can be gained in the accurate way. To find the more accurate value there are more normalization techniques are available. In this research method min-max normalization technique is utilized for the accurate finding of missing values. It is used to find the boundary range for the missing value data. The algorithm is given as follows:

Algorithm 1: Missing Value Handling with K Means Algorithm

Input: Dataset with missing values

Output: Missing values filled clusters

1. Initialize clustering

2. Find the maximum and minimum range of each feature present in the dataset

3. Find the missing value using Max and Min range values using following equation

$$v' = \frac{v - \min(e)}{\max(e) - \min(e)}$$

4. Calculate the average score of each data point.

   1) di= x1, x2,x3,x4…xn

   2) di(avg)=(w1*x1+w2*x2+w3*x3+…..wm*xm)/m where x= attribute's value, m= no of attributes, w= weight to multiply to ensure fair distribution of cluster.

5. Calculate mean values

6. Replace missing values

The above algorithm can replace the missing values present in the dataset gathered based on which accurate prediction can be done. After missing value replacement, feature reduction is done which is explained in the following sub section.

3.3.2. Feature Reduction Using Fuzzy Based Rough Set Theory

Presence of the irrelevant information present in the database would lead to inaccurate prediction outcome and also would cause more computational complexity. For the accurate prediction outcome, it is required to remove the irrelevant information present in the dataset. In the proposed research method fuzzy rough set theory is utilized to select the more relevant data information which would remove the irrelevant information's. Thus the heart disease prediction outcome can be optimized.

The main goal of fuzzy rough set theory is to find the relevant data's by avoiding the irrelevant information present in the database and to present small volume of dataset. The fuzzy rough set theory is based on the equivalence relationship present between the multiple objects present in the database. In order to tackle the uncertainty problem this work attempts to derive the structural characteristics similarity present between multiple objects. Here fuzzy relationship is derived in the numerical representation format. These fuzzy relations are utilized then to derive the fuzzy rough set which would include only relevant features.

There are two types of fuzzy relations are considered in this work for generating the fuzzy based rough set. Those are multiplicative preference relations and fuzzy preference relations. For example consider U as nonempty universe and R as a fuzzy relation factor. The minimum and maximum bound values of fuzzy can be calculated as

(1) S-lower approximation operator: $\underline{R_S A(x)} = \inf_{u \leftarrow U} S\,(N(R(x, u)), A(u))$

(2) T-upper approximation operator: $\overline{R_T}A(x) = \sup_{u \leftarrow U} T(R(x, u), A(u))$

(3) θ-lower approximation operator: $\underline{R_\theta}A(x) = \inf_{u \leftarrow U} \theta(R(x, u), A(u))$

(4) σ-upper approximation operator: $\overline{R_\sigma}A(x) = \sup_{u \leftarrow U} T(N(x, u), A(u))$

Where S, T, θ and σ are mapping functions which is used to establish the relationship between the structural characteristics of attributes present in the database. The mail goal of this research method is to establish the relationship between attributes to remove the irrelevant data which is achieved in this research method.

Fuzzy preference relation R is defined as the fuzzy product set U×U which is a product relation between the nonempty universe data. This relationship can be represented as a membership function$\mu_R: U \times U \rightarrow [0,1]$. Here it can be assumed U as finite dataset for which relationship degree is measured as absolute product operation outcome.

Input: Decision table S = (CDUDT)

Output: One feature subset sub

Step 1: sub ← ∅, RS_1 ← sub, P_1 ← {RS_1} and US_1 ← U;// sub is the pool to conserve the selected attributes

Step 2: While EvalF (sub, DT) ≠ EvalF (CD, DT)

Do

{

Compute the positive region of forward approximation $POT_{P_i}^{U}(DT)$

US_{i+1} ←US- $POT_{P_i}^{U}(DT)$ //Remaining sets in the universal set

A ← c − sub;

Select $a_0 \in$ A which satisfies Sig (a_0, sub, DT, US_i)=max {Sig (a_0, sub, DT, US_i), $a_k \in$ A},

If

{

Sig (a_0, sub, DT, US_i) > 0;

then sub← sub ∪ {a_0},

}

Else

{

$RS_i \leftarrow RS_i \cup \{a_0\}$;

$PO_i \leftarrow \{RS_1, RS_2, \ldots, RS_i\}$;

}

Step 3: Return sub and end

3.3.3. Optimal Feature Selection Using Improved Bee Colony Approach

Heart disease outcome purely depends on the types of features given to the training process. The risk factors of heart disease given to training process would increase the prediction accuracy and also it can be processed with reduced time complexity. Thus it is required to select the risk factors from the database, which can predict the heart disease in the accurate manner. In this research method Improved Bee Colony Approach is utilized for the optimal risk factor selection.

Artificial Bee colony Algorithm: Artificial bee colony algorithm (ABC), proposed by Karaboga in 2005 for real-parameter optimization, is a recently introduced optimization algorithm which simulates the foraging behavior of a bee colony. ABC classifies the foraging artificial bees into three groups, namely, employed bees, onlooker bees and scout bees. Half of the colony consists of employed bees, and the other half includes onlooker bees. Employed bees search the food around the food source in their memory; meanwhile they pass their food information to onlooker bees. Onlooker bees tend to select good food sources from those founded by the employed bees, and then further search the foods around the selected food source. Scout bees are translated from a few employed bees, which abandon their food sources and search new ones. Similar to the other population-based algorithms, ABC is an iterative process. The units of the basic ABC can be explained as follows:

Initialization of the population: The initial population of solutions is filled with SN number of randomly generated n-dimensional real-valued vectors (i.e., food sources). Let $X_i = \{x_{i,1}, x_{i,2}, \ldots, x_{i,n}\}$ represent the ith food source in the population, and then each food source is generated as in equation 3.1:

$$x_{i,j} = x_{min,j} + rand\,(0,1)(x_{max,j} - x_{min,j}) \tag{3.1}$$

where i = 1,2, ,SN, j = 1,2, ,n. $x_{min,j}$ and $x_{max,j}$ are the lower and upper bounds for the dimension j, respectively. These food sources are randomly assigned to SN number of employed bees and their fit nesses are evaluated.

Initialization of the bee phase: At this stage, each employed bee X_i generates a new food source V_i in the neighborhood of its present position by using solution search equation as in equation 3.2:

$$v_{i,j} = x_{i,j} + \Phi_{i,j}\,(x_{i,j}-x_{k,j}) \tag{3.2}$$

where k ∈ {1,2, ,SN} and j∈{1,2, ,n} are randomly chosen indexes; k has to be different from i; $f_{i,j}$ is a random number in the range [1, 1]. Once V_i is obtained, it will be evaluated and compared to X_i. If the fitness of V_i is equal to or better than that of X_i, V_i will replace X_i and become a new member of the population; otherwise X_i is retained. In other words, a greedy selection mechanism is employed between the old and candidate solutions.

Calculating probability values involved in probabilistic selection: After all employed bees complete their searches, they share their information related to the nectar amounts and the positions of their sources with the onlooker bees on the dance area. An onlooker bee evaluates the nectar information taken from all employed bees and chooses a food source site with a probability related to its nectar amount. This probabilistic selection depends on the fitness values of the solutions in the population. A fitness based selection scheme might be a roulette wheel, ranking based, stochastic universal sampling, tournament selection or another selection scheme. In basic ABC, roulette wheel selection scheme in which each slice is proportional in size to the fitness value is employed as in equation 3.3:

$$p_i = {f_i}/{\sum_{j=1}^{SN} f_i} \tag{3.3}$$

where f_i is the fitness value of solution i. Obviously, the higher the f_i is, the more probability that the ith food source is selected.

Onlooker bee phase: An onlooker bee evaluates the nectar information taken from all the employed bees and selects a food source X_i depending on its probability value p_i. Once the onlooker has selected her food source X_i, she produces a modification on X_i by using Eq. (2.2). As in the case of the employed bees, if the modified food source has a better or equal nectar amount than X_i, the modified food source will replace X_i and become a new member in the population.

Scout bee phase: If a food source X_i cannot be further improved through a predetermined number of trials limit, the food source is assumed to be abandoned, and the corresponding employed bee becomes a scout. The scout produces a food source randomly as in equation 3.4:

$$x_{i,j} = x_{min,j} + \text{rand}\ (0,1)(x_{max,j} - x_{min,j}) \tag{3.4}$$

Where j=1,2,…,n

Algorithm 1: Artificial bee colony algorithm

1. Initialize the population of solutions $x_{i,j}$, i = 1,2,…,SN, j = 1,2,…,n, $trial_i = 0$, $trial_i = 0$ is the non-improvement number of the solution X_i, used for abandonment

2. Evaluate the population

3. cycle = 1

4. repeat

5. {– – Produce a new food source population for employed bees – –}

6. for i = 1 to SN do

7. Produce a new food source V_i for the employed bee of the food source X_i using (2.2) and evaluate its quality

8. Apply a greedy selection process between V_i and X_i and select the better one

9. If solution X_i does not improve $trial_i = trial_i + 1$, otherwise $trial_i = 0$

10. end for

11: Calculate the probability values p_i by (2.3) for the solutions using fitness values

{– – Produce a new food source population for onlooker bees – –}

t = 0, i = 1

repeat

if random < p_i then

Produce a new V_i food source by (2.2) for onlooker bee

Apply a greedy selection process between V_i and X_i and select the better one

If solution X_i does not improve $trial_i = trial_i + 1$, otherwise $trial_i = 0$

t = t+1

end if

until (t=SN)

{– – Determine Scout – –}

if max($trial_i$)>limit then

Replace X_i with a new randomly produced solution by (2.4)

end if

Memorize the best solution achieved so far

cycle = cycle+1

until (cycle=Maximum Cycle Number)

By using the above equation most solution optimal set of risk factors would be identified.

Improved Bee colony Algorithm: It is clear that ABC/best/1 has a good capacity of the exploitation. Unfortunately, ABC/best/1 can reduce the exploration of ABC. If all bees produce new food sources, the algorithm can easily get trapped in the local optima when solving complex multimodal problems. In other words, ABC which is good at exploration but poor at exploitation results in a slow convergence. While ABC/best/1, which is good at exploitation but poor at exploration, cannot avoid premature convergence. To address this contradiction, we propose the new search mechanism which introduces the selective probability P to balance the exploration of the solution and the exploitation of the modified solution search. Based on the above explanation, the pseudo-code of IABC is given below:

Algorithm 3: Modified artificial bee colony algorithm

1. Set the population size SN, give the maximum number of function evaluations, Max.FE

2. Create an initial population $\{X_i| \ i = 1,2, ,SN\}$, calculate the function values of the population $\{f_i|i = 1,2, ,SN\}$

3. While (stopping criterion is not met, namely FE < Max.FE) do

4. for i = 1 to SN do

5. {– – Produce a new food source using the new search mechanism– –}

6. Choose X_{r1}, X_{r2} randomly from the current population, the indices r_1, r_2 are mutually exclusive integers randomly chosen from the range [1, SN], which are also different from the index i

7. Randomly choose j from {1,2, ,n} and produce $\Phi_{i,j} \in [-1.1]$

8. Generate a new food source V_i according to Equation 3.5

$$V_{i,j} = X_{best,j} + \Phi_{i,j} \ (X_{r1,j} - X_{r2,j}) \tag{3.5}$$

9. if $f(V_i) < f(X_i)$ then

10. $X_i = V_i$

11. else then

12. if rand(0,1)<P then

14. Randomly choose j from {1,2, ,n}, k∈{1,2, ,SN} which has to be different from i and produce $\Phi_{i,j} \in [-1,1]$

15. Generate a new food source V_i according to Equation 3.6

$$v_{i,j} = x_{i,j} + fi,j\ \Phi_{i,j}\ (x_{i,j} - x_{k,j}) \tag{3.6}$$

16. if $f(V_i) < f(X_i)$ then

17. $X_i = V_i$

18. end if

19. end if

20. end if

21. end for

22. end while (FE = Max.FE)

3.3.4. Optimal Heart Disease Prediction Using Support Vector Machine

After prediction optimal set of risk factors, those values would be learned in order to make more reliable and optimal prediction outcome. In this research method SVM classifier is utilized for the optimal prediction of heart disease. A Support Vector Machine (SVM) is a discriminative classifier formally defined by a separating hyper plane. In other words, given labeled training data (supervised learning), the algorithm outputs an optimal hyper plane which categorizes new examples.

SVM is supervised learning models with associated learning algorithms that analyze data and recognize patterns, used for classification and regression analysis. Support Vector Machines are based on the concept of decision planes that define decision boundaries. A decision plane is one that separates between a set of objects having different class memberships.

A schematic example is shown in the illustration below in figure 3.4. In this example, the objects belong either to class GREEN or RED. The separating line defines a boundary on the right side of which all objects are GREEN and to the left of which all objects are RED. Any new object (white circle) falling to the right is labeled, i.e., classified, as GREEN (or classified as RED should it fall to the left of the separating line).

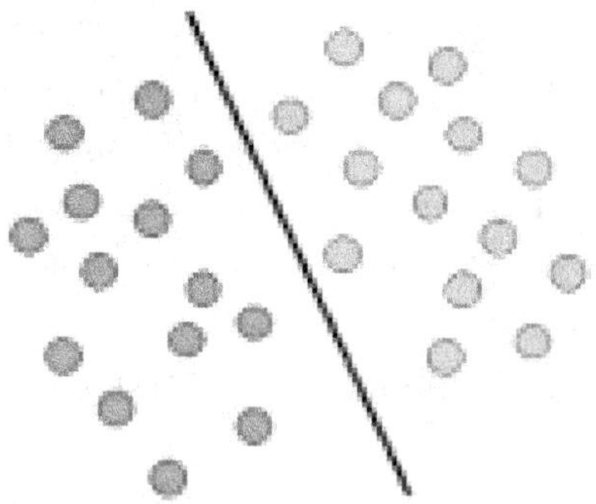

Figure 3.4. Schematic example of linear classification

The above is a classic example of a linear classifier, i.e., a classifier that separates a set of objects into their respective groups (GREEN and RED in this case) with a line. Most classification tasks, however, are not that simple, and often more complex structures are needed in order to make an optimal separation, i.e., correctly classify new objects (test cases) on the basis of the examples that are available (train cases).

This situation is depicted in the illustration below in figure 3.5. Compared to the previous schematic, it is clear that a full separation of the GREEN and RED objects would require a curve (which is more complex than a line). Classification tasks based on drawing separating lines to distinguish between objects of different class memberships are known as hyper plane classifiers. Support Vector Machines are particularly suited to handle such tasks.

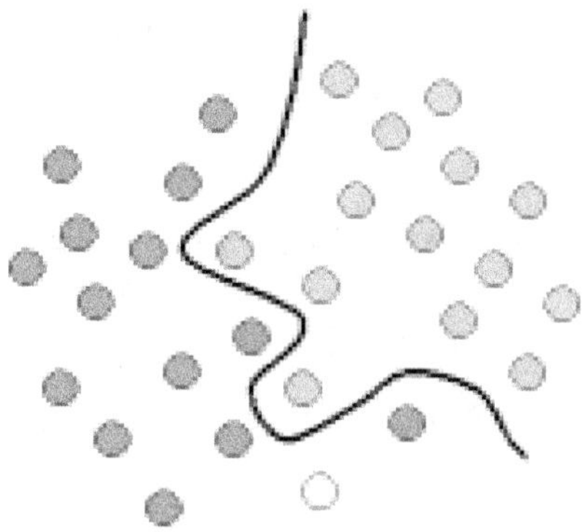

Figure 3.5. Schematic examples of non linear classifier

The illustration below in figure 3.6 shows the basic idea behind Support Vector Machines. Here we see the original objects (left side of the schematic) mapped, i.e., rearranged, using a set of mathematical functions, known as kernels. The process of rearranging the objects is known as mapping (transformation). Note that in this new setting, the mapped objects (right side of the schematic) is linearly separable and, thus, instead of constructing the complex curve (left schematic), all we have to do is to find an optimal line that can separate the GREEN and the RED objects.

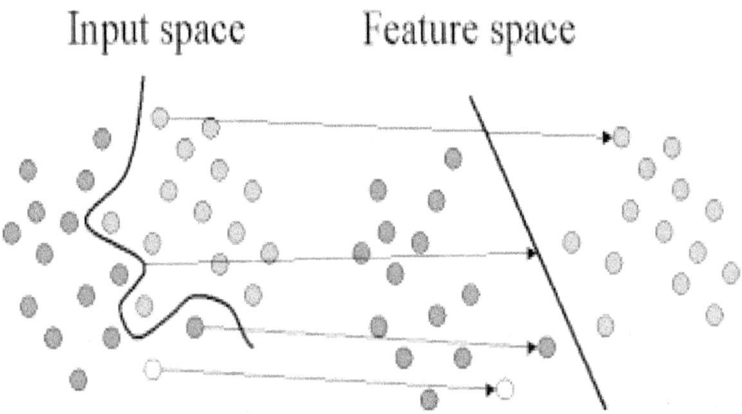

Figure 3.6. Basic functioning of support vector machine

Given a set of training examples, each marked for belonging to one of two categories, an SVM training algorithm builds a model that assigns new examples into one category or the other.

Formula

To reduce the error minimization we can use given below Equation 3.7

$$\Phi(w) = \frac{1}{2}||w||^2 \quad (3.7)$$

Estimating function is given in Equation 3.8

$$F(x) = \sum_{i=1}^{nsv}(x_i, y_i) \quad (3.8)$$

Algorithm

Given dataset X=(x1, y1),……,(xn, yn), C // x and y –labeled sequence and C-class

Initialize vector v=0, b=0; class // v-vector and b-bias

Train an initial SVM

For each $x_i \in X$ do // xi is a vector containing features describing example i

Classify x_i using $f(x_i)$

If $y_i f(x_i) < 1$ // prediction class label

Find w', b' for known data // w', b' for new data

Add x_i to known data

If the prediction is wrong then retrain

Repeat

End

Error values are minimized using equation (1)

Classify results using equation (2)

3.4. RESULTS AND DISCUSSION

The experiments are conducted in the mat lab simulation environment where the performance evaluation between the proposed method namely Heart disease prediction using Fuzzy Rough Set Theory combined with Support Vector Machine (FRS - SVM) and the existing methods namely Coronary Heart Disease prediction using Particle Swarm Optimization Approach (CHD-PSO), Artificial Neural Network based Prediction (ANN) is done. The performance metrics that are considered in this research work for the comparison evaluation are, "Accuracy, Precision, Recall, F-Measure". The performance evaluation are shown and explained in the following sub sections.

3.4.1. Accuracy

Accuracy is defined as the proportion of true positives and true negatives among the total number of results obtained. Accuracy is evaluated as in Equation 3.9.

$$\text{Accuracy} = \frac{(\text{True positive} + \text{True negative})}{(\text{True positive} + \text{True negative} + \text{False positive} + \text{False negative})} \quad (3.9)$$

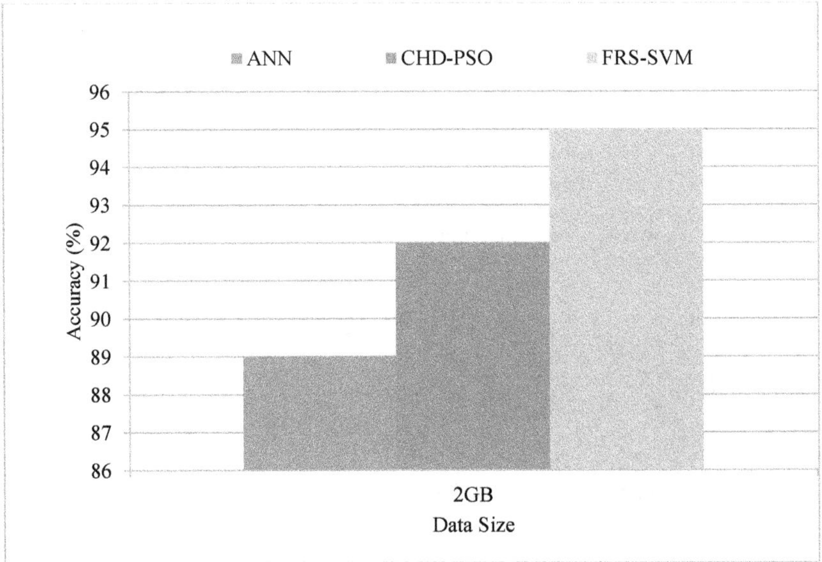

Figure 3.7. Accuracy comparison graph

From the above graph mentioned in (Figure-3.7), it is proved that the proposed method namely FRS-SVM can provide better performance result than the existing research methodologies. From the analytical evaluation of the results, it can be proved that the proposed methodology FRS-SVM shows 6% better than CHD-PSO, 14% better performance than ANN method.

3.4.2. Precision

Precision value is evaluated according to the relevant information at true positive prediction, false positive. The precision calculation procedure is given in following Equation 3.10.

$$\text{Precision} = \frac{\text{True Positive}}{(\text{True Positive} + \text{False Positive})} \quad (3.10)$$

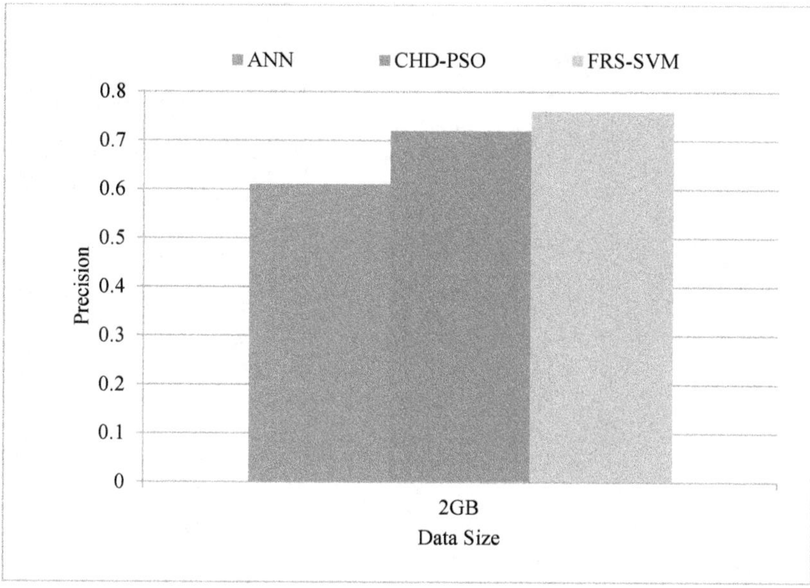

Figure 3.8. Precision comparison graph

From the above graph it is proved that the proposed method namely FRS-SVM can provide better performance result than the existing research methodologies in terms of precision. From the analytical evaluation of the results, it can be proved that the proposed methodology FRS-SVM shows 13% better than ANN, 17% better performance than CHD-PSO method.

3.4.3. Recall

Recall value is evaluated according to the retrieval of information at true positive prediction, false negative. Recall evaluation is shown in following Equation 3.11.

$$\text{Recall} = \frac{\text{True Positive}}{(\text{True positive} + \text{False negative})} \tag{3.11}$$

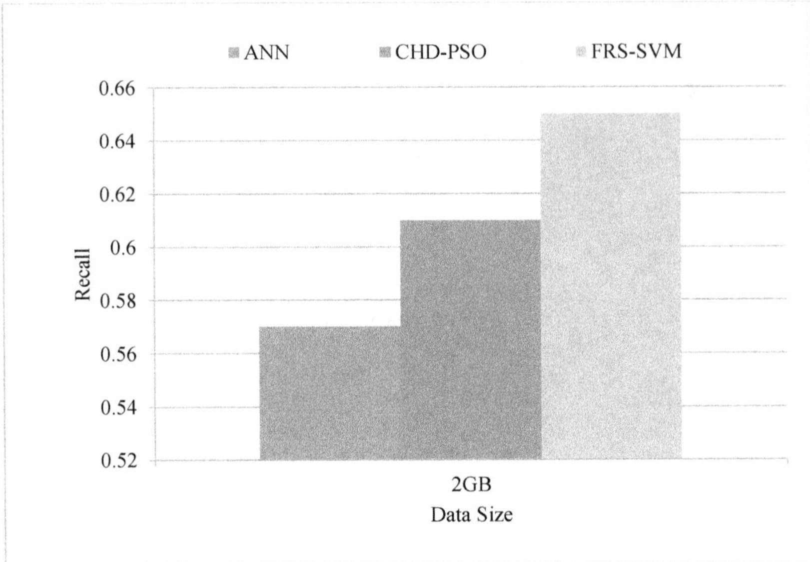

Figure 3.9. Recall comparison graph

From the above graph it is proved that the proposed method namely FRS-SVM can provide better performance result than the existing research methodologies. From the analytical evaluation of the results, it can be proved that the proposed methodology FRS-SVM shows 17% better performance than CHD-PSO, 25% better performance than ANN method.

3.4.4. F-Measure

The F-Measure computes some average of the information retrieval precision and recall metrics. It is measured as like in Equation 3.12.

$$\mathrm{F-Measure} = \frac{2 * \mathrm{precision.recall}}{\mathrm{precision} + \mathrm{recall}} \tag{3.12}$$

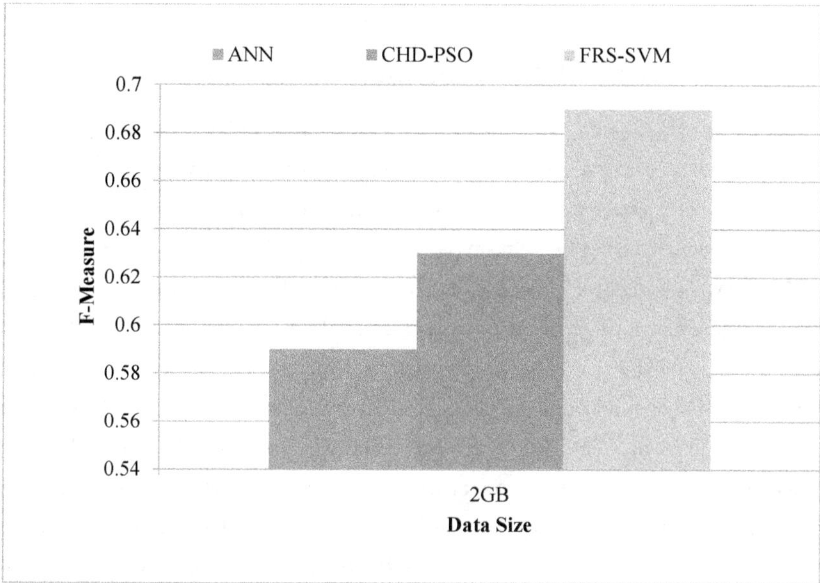

Figure 3.10. F-measure comparison graph

From the above graph it is proved that the proposed method namely FRS-SVM can provide better performance result than the existing research methodologies. From the analytical evaluation of the results, it can be proved that the proposed methodology FRS-SVM shows 16% better than CHD-PSO, 23% better performance than ANN method.

3.5. SUMMARY

In this work, initially Pre-processing is done by using K-means clustering Algorithm to make the dataset cleaner, consistent and noise free. Then Feature reduction of the dataset is done by using Fuzzy based rough set theory. The fuzzy rough sets extend the rough set concept through the use of fuzzy equivalence classes. From this reduced feature set, optimal feature selection is done by using Improved Bee Colony approach. Finally, classification of dataset is done by using Support vector machine. The overall evaluation of the proposed research methodology is done by using the Mat lab simulation environment from which it is proved that the proposed work namely NORFS-HDPS can lead to optimal outcome than the existing research techniques.

CHAPTER 4

ACCURATE HEART DISEASE PREDICTION SYSTEM

Heart disease is the most common found disease in various peoples which would cause more serious and dangerous effects. There is various research methods has been proposed earlier whose main goal is to predict the heart disease more accurately. In our previous research method Fuzzy Rough Set Theory combined with Support Vector Machine (FRS - SVM) is introduced which can ensures the optimal prediction rate by selecting the risk factors accurately which can lead to improved accuracy rate. However FRS-SVM might lack in its performance in case of presence of more missing values in the database. This research method cannot support the large dimensional dataset which needs to be focused well enough for accurate prediction rate. This problem is resolved in the proposed research method by introducing the framework namely Heart disease prediction using Alpha Rough Set Theory combined with Fuzzy SVM (ARST-FSVM). In this research method, Modified K-Means clustering algorithm is used for preprocessing the input dataset which would avoid the noisy data present in the database. Then missing data value in the database is handled using normalization technique where NLLS imputation is applied. And then feature dimensionality reduction is done using Alpha rough set theory (α-RST) approach. From those reduced feature set, optimal feature selection in terms of relevancy is done using Hybrid Bee colony algorithm with Glowworm Swarm Optimization (HBC-GSO) approach. Finally heart disease prediction is done using classifier namely fuzzy based SVM.

4.1. INTRODUCTION

Heart disease is the most common and frequently identified disease over people which would cause more serious effects (Kaur and Kaur, 2016). Treating and curing heart disease is the most complex process that might cause sudden death. This can be solved by predicting the heart disease earlier, so that patients can be treated before serious causes. There are various research method has been introduced earlier that focus on earlier diagnosis of heart disease occurrence (Joshi and Nair, 2015). Those research method analysis the history of information about the patients for treating them. However research method required complete knowledge about the patients which is not possibly applicable in the real world to gather complete information (Kaur and Singh, 2014).

And also existing research methods may not produce accurate outcomes, since it only considers limited information to learn and derive the outcome. Limited information would lead to reduced prediction accuracy which needs to be concentrated more for the earlier diagnosis of heart disease (Lemke and Mueller, 2003). There are numerous research has been introduced earlier for the earlier prediction of heart disease occurrence. Data mining techniques includes statistical analysis, machine learning techniques and database techniques are used to predict the disease occurrence by analyzing and finding the patterns. Based on these patterns, accurate disease diagnosis can be ensured (Thanigaivel and Kumar, 2015).

By adapting these techniques heart disease prediction can be done accurately by analyzing and learning characteristics and structural behavior of heart disease dataset (Gudadhe et al., 2010). There are variety of soft computing techniques are available earlier which attempts to predict the heart disease occurrence. Those techniques can learn and provide the accurate heart disease outcome by learning and providing the data base patterns.

This problem is resolved in the proposed research method by introducing the framework namely Heart disease prediction using Alpha Rough Set Theory combined with Fuzzy SVM (ARST-FSVM). In this research method, Modified K-Means clustering algorithm is used for preprocessing the input dataset which would avoid the noisy data present in the database. Then missing data value in the database is handled using normalization technique where NLLS imputation is applied. And then feature dimensionality reduction is done using Alpha rough set theory (α-RST) approach. From those reduced feature set, optimal feature selection in terms of relevancy is done using Hybrid Bee colony algorithm with Glowworm Swarm Optimization (HBC-GSO) approach. Finally heart disease prediction is done using classifier namely fuzzy based SVM.

4.2. EARLY DIAGNOSIS OF HEART DISEASE BY USING OPTIMAL RISK FACTOR SELECTION

Heart disease prediction is the most important task in the medical field whose main goal is to detect the heart disease occurrence on patients earlier, so that proper and immediate treatment can be provide before dangerous causes. This is ensured in the proposed research method by introducing the novel research technique namely Alpha Rough Set Theory combined with Fuzzy SVM (ARST-FSVM). In this research method, Modified K-Means clustering algorithm is used for preprocessing the input dataset which would avoid the noisy data present in the database. Then missing data value in the database is handled using normalization technique where NLLS imputation is applied. And then feature dimensionality reduction is done using Alpha rough set theory (α-RST) approach. From those reduced feature set, optimal feature selection in terms of relevancy is done using Hybrid Bee colony algorithm with Glowworm Swarm Optimization (HBC-GSO) approach. Finally heart disease prediction is done using classifier namely fuzzy based SVM. The detailed explanation of the proposed research methodology has been given in the following sub sections.

4.3. PREPROCESSING USING MODIFIED K-MEANS ALGORITHM

Preprocessing and Feature Selection- involves choosing an appropriate feature, and doing appropriate preprocessing and feature extraction on data items to measure the values of the chosen feature set. It will often be desirable to choose a subset of all the features available, to reduce the dimensionality of the problem space. This step often requires a good deal of domain knowledge and data analysis. Clustering Algorithm- which uses particular similarity measures as subroutines. The particular choice of clustering algorithms depends on the desired properties of the final clustering. A clustering algorithm attempts to find natural groups of components (or data) based on some similarity and also finds the centroid of a group of data sets. To determine cluster membership, most algorithms evaluate the distance between a point and the cluster centroids. The output from a clustering algorithm is basically a statistical description of the cluster centroids with the number of components in each cluster.

K-Means (KM) is considered one of the major algorithms widely used in clustering. However, it still has some problems, and one of them is in its initialization step where it is normally performed randomly. Another problem for KM is that it converges to local minima. In the enhanced clustering method discussed in this thesis, both the phases of the original k-means algorithm are modified to improve the accuracy and efficiency. The enhanced method is outlined as below.

Algorithm 1: The enhanced method

Input:D = {d1, d2,......,dn} // set of n data items

k // Number of desired clusters

Output: A set of k clusters.

Steps:

1. Phase 1: Determine the initial centroids of the clusters by using Algorithm 2.

2. Phase 2: Assign each data point to the appropriate clusters.

In the first phase, the initial centroids are determined systematically so as to produce clusters with better accuracy. The second phase data points are assigned to appropriate clusters. It starts by forming the initial clusters based on the relative distance of each data-point from the initial centroids. These clusters are subsequently fine-tuned by using a heuristic

Algorithm 2: Finding the initial centroids

Input: D = {d1, d2,......,dn} // set of n data items

k // Number of desired clusters

Output: A set of k initial centroids.

Steps:

1. Set m = 1;

2. Compute the distance between each data point and all other data- points in the set D;

3. Find the closest pair of data points from the set D and form a data-point set Am (1<= m <= k) which contains these two data- points, Delete these two data points from the set D;

4. Find the data point in D that is closest to the data point set Am, Add it to Am and delete it from D;

5. Repeat step 4 until the number of data points in Am reaches 0.75*(n/k);

6. If m<=m<=k) find the arithmetic mean of the vectors of data points in Am, these means will be the initial centroids.

Algorithm 2 describes the method for finding initial centroids of the clusters. Initially, compute the distances between each data point and all other data points in the set of data points. Then find out the closest pair of data points and form a set A1 consisting of these two data points, and delete them from the data point set D. Then determine the data point which is closest to the set A1, add it to A1 and delete it from D. Repeat this procedure until the number of elements in the set A1 reaches a threshold. At that point go back to the second step and form another data-point set A2. Repeat this till " k" such sets of data points are obtained. Finally the initial centroids are obtained by averaging all the vectors in each data-point set. The Euclidean distance is used for determining the closeness of each data point to the cluster centroids.

4.4. MISSING VALUE REPLACEMENT USING NLLS IMPUTATION METHOD

In statistics, imputation is the process of replacing missing data with substituted values. When substituting for a data point, it is known as "unit imputation"; when substituting for a component of a data point, it is known as "item imputation". There are three main problems that missing data causes: missing data can introduce a substantial amount of bias, make the handling and analysis of the data more arduous, and create reductions in efficiency. Because missing data can create problems for analyzing data, imputation is seen as a way to avoid pitfalls involved with list wise deletion of cases that have missing values. That is to say, when one or more values are missing for a case, most statistical packages default to discarding any case that has a missing value, which may introduce bias or affect the representativeness of the results.

In order to deal with the problem of increased noise due to imputation, Rubin (1987) developed a method for averaging the outcomes across multiple imputed data sets to account for this. All multiple imputation methods follow three steps.

1. Imputation - Similar to single imputation, missing values are imputed. However, the imputed values are drawn *m* times from a distribution rather than just once. At the end of this step, there should be *m* completed datasets.
2. Analysis - Each of the *m* datasets is analyzed. At the end of this step there should be *m* analyses.
3. Pooling - The *m* results are consolidated into one result by calculating the mean, variance, and confidence interval of the variable of concern.

Just as there are multiple methods of single imputation, there are multiple methods of multiple imputations as well. One advantage that multiple imputations has over the single imputation and complete case methods is that, multiple imputation is flexible and can be used in a wide variety of scenarios. Multiple imputations can be used in cases where the data is missing completely, missing at random, and even when the data is missing not at random. However, the primary method of multiple imputations is Multiple Imputation by Chained Equations (MICE). It is also known as "fully conditional specification" and, "sequential regression multiple imputation." An important thing to note is that MICE should be implemented only when the missing data follow the missing at random mechanism.

As illustrated in the previous section, single imputation does not take into account the uncertainty in the imputations. After imputation, the data is treated as if they were the actual real values in single imputation. The negligence of uncertainty in the imputation can and will lead to overly precise results and errors in any conclusions drawn. By imputing multiple times, multiple imputations certainly accounts for the uncertainty and range of values that the true value could have taken.

Additionally, while it is the case that singles imputation and complete case are easier to implement, multiple imputation is not very difficult to implement. There are a wide range of different statistical packages in different statistical software that readily allow someone to perform multiple imputations. For example, the MICE package allows users in R to perform multiple imputations using the MICE method.

Imputation preserves all cases by replacing missing data with an estimated value based on other available information. Once all missing values have been imputed, the data set can then be analyzed using standard techniques for complete data. Imputation theory is constantly developing and thus requires consistent attention to new information regarding the subject. There have been many theories embraced by scientists to account for missing data but the majority of them introduce large amounts of bias. A few of the well known attempts to deal with missing data include: hot deck and cold deck imputation; list wise and pair wise deletion; mean imputation; regression imputation; last observation carried forward; stochastic imputation; and multiple imputation.

In this proposed work a New Local Least Square imputation based algorithm (NLLS impute) implemented. This algorithm is most as K-nearest neighbour imputation algorithm. In this proposal work to select the K-nearest data from the complete set of obtained candidate gene as a substitute of the complete dataset and also reuse the imputed information available obtained. For this method the larger amount of information available for estimating its missing values in the target data. Subsequently the highest missing rate will be imputed in the target data with the available information. It means the imputed information obtained from the data's whose missing values have been imputed before. The New Local Least Square impute algorithm proceeds as follows:

Algorithm: NSLLS impute

Input: The m number of data's and n number of samples, T it contains some artificial missing entries.

Output: The missing entries are predicted.

1. At first from the complete data matrix X to replace the missing positions of the given data matrix.
2. According to their missing rate and imputation one after another the m numbers of data's in X are sorted in ascending order.
3. For each target data in X do:
   a) For each missing position p in target data do:
      i) The Pearson Correlation coefficient is used to select the k number of candidate data nearest to the target data. For the period of the computation of Pearson Correlation coefficient the missing positions filled with row average are ignored.
      ii) The conception of local least squares is imputing the missing position p in the target data beneath deliberation Perez-Bellido et al. (2008).
      iii) The result of imputed values is positioned in the missing positions of the considered target data.
4. End

4.5. FEATURE REDUCTION USING ALPHA ROUGH SET THEORY

Pawlak's rough set model can only deal with data sets with discrete values. However, the real-world applications usually contain real-valued attributes. Thus, the Alpha-rough set model has been proposed to deal with this case. An illustrative example is given to represent the computing procedure of the proposed algorithm.

4.5.1. Generalized Information System

Let U be a finite set of objects or examples, U = $\{x_1, x_2, \ldots, x_n\}$. These objects of the universe U are characterized by a finite set of attributes, denoted as Q . fq1; q2; . . . ; qmg. An attribute qi may be qualitative or quantitative. A qualitative attribute q_i has a domain v_{qi} which determines the set of possible values for attribute q_i. For instance, the attribute Age may be seen as a qualitative attribute (nominal or categorical) which is defined by its discrete domain (a finite discrete set) as {young, adult, middle_age, old, too_old}. Equivalently, each value of Age is described by its membership function.

The attribute Age may also be seen as a quantitative (cardinal) one, which is defined by its continuous domain (interval) as [a, b]. A preprocessing discretization phase is generally necessary for a numerical attribute to divide its domain into intervals which correspond to qualitative terms. This translation process may be performed automatically [discretization] or by an expert. Membership function which represents the value middle_age of attribute Age. It assumes that concepts are crisp, i.e., the age of a person is middle_age or is not. This approach is based on 2-valued logic ± black or white. Consider next that middle_age is defined by fuzzy property ``around 45 years''. Qualitative attributes may be interpreted as linguistic variables, according to the fuzzy set theory. In this case, there is not a unique membership function for middle_age and the expert has to determine it according to the nature of the application domain.

4.5.2. Information Measures for Fuzzy-Rough Set Model

A fuzzy equivalence relation would be generated by a real valued attribute, instead of crisp equivalence relation. A crisp rough equivalence relation is central to crisp rough sets, while the fuzzy equivalence relation is central to fuzzy rough sets. $\widetilde{R}$ is a fuzzy equivalence relation if $\widetilde{R}$ satisfies

(1) Reflectivity : $\widetilde{R}(x, x) = 1, \forall x \in X$

(2) Symmetry: $\widetilde{R}(x, y) = \widetilde{R}(y, x), \forall x, y \in X$

(3) Transitivity : $\widetilde{R}(x, z) \geq \min_{y}\{\widetilde{R}(x, y), \widetilde{R}(y, z)\}$

Given a non-empty finite set X, $\widetilde{R}$ is a fuzzy equivalence relation defined on X, denoted by a relation matrix $M(\widetilde{R})$ as in Equation 4.1:

$$M(\widetilde{R}) = \begin{pmatrix} r_{11} & r_{12} & \cdots & r_{1n} \\ r_{21} & r_{22} & \cdots & r_{2n} \\ \cdots & \cdots & \cdots & \cdots \\ r_{n1} & r_{n2} & \cdots & r_{nn} \end{pmatrix} \quad (4.1)$$

Where $r_{ij} \in [0, 1]$is the relation value of x_i and x_j, which can also be written as $\widetilde{R}(x_i, x_j)$, where $x_i, x_j \in X$. For the crisp rough set model, $r_{ij} = 1$ if x_i equals to x_j with respect to the crisp equivalence relation R; otherwise, $r_{ij} = 0$.

Algorithm 3.

Step 1. Let B =∅;

Step 2. For every attribute a ∈ C - B, compute the significance of condition attribute a, $\widetilde{Gain}$(a, B, D);

Step 3. Select the attribute which maximize the $\widetilde{Gain}$(a, B, D); record it as a;

Step 4. If $\widetilde{Gain}$(a, B, D) > 0, then B ← B ∪ {a}, go to Step 2, else go to Step 5;

Step 5. The set B is the selected attributes

4.5.3. Dependency and Reduction

In rough set theory, we say that a set of attributes R depends on a set of attributes P, denoted P → R, iff all elementary sets of the indiscernibility relation associated with P are subsets of some elementary sets defined by R. A set attributes may be reduced in such a way that the resulting set of attributes, which is smaller, provides the same quality of classification as the original set of attributes. This means that elementary sets generated by the reduced set A are identical to those generated by the original set of attributes P, i.e., IND (A) = IND (P). The smallest reduced set of P is called a reduct. In the case where an information system has more than one reduct, the intersection of these reducts is computed. It is called the core and represents the most significant attributes in the system.

4.6. OPTIMAL FEATURE SELECTION USING HYBRID BEE COLONY-GLOWWORM SWARM APPROACH

Optimal feature selection plays a greatest role in the prediction technology which attempts to select the more relevant features from the input dataset. This more relevant input data subset given as input to the classifier would improve the prediction outcome. Feature selection allows the reduction of feature space, which is crucial in reducing the training time and improving the prediction accuracy. This is achieved by removing irrelevant, redundant, and noisy features (i.e., selecting the subset of features that can achieve the best performance in terms of accuracy and computational time). In this research work, hybrid bee colony Glow worm swarm optimization algorithm is introduced. In this method initially relevant feature subset based on correlation is selected using Bee colony algorithm whose outcome is given as input to the glowworm swarm optimization approach. This method would result the most optimal feature subset which would improve the final prediction outcome.

4.6.1. Bee Colony Algorithm

Artificial bee colony algorithm (ABC), proposed by Karaboga in 2005 for real-parameter optimization, is a recently introduced optimization algorithm which simulates the foraging behavior of a bee colony. ABC classifies the foraging artificial bees into three groups, namely, employed bees, onlooker bees and scout bees. Half of the colony consists of employed bees, and the other half includes onlooker bees. Employed bees search the food around the food source in their memory; meanwhile they pass their food information to onlooker bees. Onlooker bees tend to select good food sources from those founded by the employed bees, and then further search the foods around the selected food source. Scout bees are translated from a few employed bees, which abandon their food sources and search new ones. Similar to the other population-based algorithms, ABC is an iterative process. The units of the basic ABC can be explained as follows:

Initialization of the population: The initial population of solutions is filled with SN number of randomly generated n-dimensional real-valued vectors (i.e., food sources). Let $X_i = \{x_{i,1}, x_{i,2}, \dots, x_{i,n}\}$ represent the ith food source in the population, and then each food source is generated as in equation 4.2:

$$x_{i,j} = x_{min,j} + \text{rand}(0,1)(x_{max,j} - x_{min,j}) \tag{4.2}$$

where i = 1,2, ,SN, j = 1,2, ,n. $x_{min,j}$ and $x_{max,j}$ are the lower and upper bounds for the dimension j, respectively. These food sources are randomly assigned to SN number of employed bees and their fitnesses are evaluated.

Initialization of the bee phase: At this stage, each employed bee X_i generates a new food source V_i in the neighborhood of its present position by using solution search equation as in equation 4.3:

$$v_{i,j} = x_{i,j} + \Phi_{i,j}(x_{i,j} - x_{k,j}) \tag{4.3}$$

where k ∈ {1,2, ,SN} and j∈{1,2, ,n} are randomly chosen indexes; k has to be different from i; $f_{i,j}$ is a random number in the range [1, 1]. Once V_i is obtained, it will be evaluated and compared to X_i. If the fitness of V_i is equal to or better than that of X_i, V_i will replace X_i and become a new member of the population; otherwise X_i is retained. In other words, a greedy selection mechanism is employed between the old and candidate solutions.

Calculating probability values involved in probabilistic selection: After all employed bees complete their searches, they share their information related to the nectar amounts and the positions of their sources with the onlooker bees on the dance area. An onlooker bee evaluates the nectar information taken from all employed bees and chooses a food source site with a probability related to its nectar amount. This probabilistic selection depends on the fitness values of the solutions in the population. A fitness based selection scheme might be a roulette wheel, ranking based, stochastic universal sampling, tournament selection or another selection scheme. In basic ABC, roulette wheel selection scheme in which each slice is proportional in size to the fitness value is employed as in equation 4.4:

$$p_i = {f_i}\Big/{\textstyle\sum_{j=1}^{SN} f_i} \tag{4.4}$$

where f_i is the fitness value of solution i. Obviously, the higher the f_i is, the more probability that the ith food source is selected.

Onlooker bee phase: An onlooker bee evaluates the nectar information taken from all the employed bees and selects a food source X_i depending on its probability value p_i. Once the onlooker has selected her food source X_i, she produces a modification on X_i by using Eq. (2.2). As in the case of the employed bees, if the modified food source has a better or equal nectar amount than X_i, the modified food source will replace X_i and become a new member in the population.

Scout bee phase: If a food source X_i cannot be further improved through a predetermined number of trials limit, the food source is assumed to be abandoned, and the corresponding employed bee becomes a scout. The scout produces a food source randomly as in equation 4.5:

$$x_{i,j} = x_{min,j} + \text{rand}\,(0,1)(x_{max,j} - x_{min,j}) \tag{4.5}$$

where j=1,2,…,n

4.6.2. Glow Worm Swarm Optimization

In GSO algorithm, the glowworm is more attractive when the luciferin value is greater, which guides other glowworms to move towards it. Each glowworm has its dynamic decision space, which contains glowworms with both values of luciferin higher than itself and distance within its dynamic decision radius. Glowworm updates its location to a glowworm in its dynamic decision space in the light of probability, and then, renews its decision space radius.

Procedure of GSO: The value of luciferin is related to both the value of luciferin in the former iteration and objective function in the current iteration. Let x_i (t) represents the location of glowworm i in the t iteration, J(x(t)) denotes the value of objective function, which is transferred to the value of luciferin denotes by l_i (t) as in equation 4.6:

$$l_i(t) = (1-\rho)l_i\,(t-1) + \gamma(x_i(t)) \tag{4.6}$$

where ρ and γ are the luciferin decay constant and enhancement constant respectively. Both of them range from 0 to 1. Each glowworm has a dynamic decision space, which contains its neighbors with higher luciferin values than its own value and the distance between them within the decision space radius. N_i (t) is the set of neighborhood of glowworm i at the t iteration, given by (2). P_{ij} (t) is deemed to be the probability of glowworm i moving toward a neighbor j in the t iteration, calculated by (4.7) and (4.8)

$$N_i(t) = \{j : d_{ij}(t) < r_d^{'}(t): l_t(t) < l_j(t)\} \tag{4.7}$$

$$p_{ij}(t) = \frac{l_j(t) - l_i(t)}{\sum_{k \in N_i(t)} l_k(t) - l_i(t)} \tag{4.8}$$

where $r_d^{'}(t)$ denotes the dynamic decision space radius of glowworm i in the t iteration, and $l_i(t)$ is the luciferin value of glowworm j after the phase of probabilistic mechanism in the t iteration. Each glowworm updates its location according to (4.9)

$$x_i(t+1) = x_i(t) + s\left(\frac{x_j(t) - x_i(t)}{\|x_j(t) - x_i(t)\|}\right) \tag{4.9}$$

where s is the step-size, || || represents the Euclidean norm operator. The radius of each glowworm dynamic decision space not only depends on the current radius of dynamic decision space, but also associates with the radial range of the luciferin sensor deemed by r_s. The update rule of each glowworm dynamic decision space radius is given by Equation 4.10:

$$r_d^i\,(t+1) = \min(r_i, \max\{0, r_d^i(t) + \beta(n_i - |N_i(t)|)\}) \tag{4.10}$$

where β denotes the dynamic decision space parameter, n_t is a control parameter for neighbors in the space. $|N_i\,(t)|$ is the number of neighbors in the dynamic decision space.

4.6.3. Hybrid Bee Colony Glow Worm Swarm Optimization

In the ABC model, the colony consists of three groups of bees: employed bees, onlookers and scouts. It is assumed that there is only one artificial employed bee for each food source. In other words, the number of employed bees in the colony is equal to the number of food sources around the hive. Employed bees go to their food source and come back to hive and dance on this area. The employed bee whose food source has been abandoned becomes a scout and starts to search for finding a new food source. Onlookers watch the dances of employed bees and choose food sources depending on dances. This process is hence characterized by a positive feedback loop. For a given classification task, the problem of feature selection can be stated as follows: given the original set, F, of n features, find subset S, which consists of m features ($m < n$, $S \subset F$), such that the classification accuracy is maximized. The feature selection representation exploited by artificial bee includes the following:

n features that constitute the original set, $F = \{f_1, f_2, \ldots, f_n\}$

A number of artificial bees to search through the feature space (na bees)

τ_i, the fitness of pheromone trail associated with feature f_i , which reflects the previous knowledge about the importance of f_i .

For each bee j, a list that contains the selected feature subset, $S_j = \{s_1, \ldots., s_m\}$

We propose to use a hybrid evaluation measure that is able to estimate the overall performance of subsets as well as the local importance of features. A classification algorithm is used to estimate the performance of subsets (i.e., wrapper evaluation function). On the other hand, the local importance of a given feature is measured using the correlation based evaluation function, which is a filter evaluation function. In the first iteration, each bee will randomly choose a feature subset of m features. Only the best k subsets, $k < na$, will be used to update the fitness and influence the feature subsets of the next iteration. In the second and following iterations, each bee will start with $m - p$ features that are randomly chosen from the previously selected k -best subsets, where p is an integer that ranges between 1 and m -1. In this way, the features that constitute the best k subsets will have more chance to be present in the subsets of the next iteration. These output subsets are given as input to GSO algorithm for obtaining more optimal feature subsets.

The glowworm swarm optimization algorithm (GSO) is a kind of new method of swarm intelligence. The agents in AGSO are thought of as glowworms that carry a luminescent quantity called luciferin. Each glowworm uses an artificial equivalent to luciferin, which we will call luciferin for short in the following, to broadcast the fitness of its current location, evaluated using the objective function, to its neighbors. That is, glowworms are attracted to neighbors that glow brighter. These movement that are based only on local information and selective neighbor interactions, enable the swarm to partition into disjoint subgroups that converge to multiple optima of a given multimodal function. According to the above principles, the AGSO have used for multi-modal functions optimization, multi-modal functions with collective robotics applications, etc.

In the GSO algorithm, each solution correspond to a glowworm in the search space, and every glowworm has a fitness value decided by function of the optimization problem .Each glowworm encodes the objective function at the current location into a luciferin value. The glowworms depend on a variable neighborhood, which is bounded above by a radial sensor range, to identify their neighbors and compute their movements. Each glowworm, using a probabilistic mechanism, selects a neighbor that has a luciferin value higher than its own and moves toward it.

A set of n glowworms are randomly deployed in a m -dimensional workspace. According to the similarity of luciferin value, divide the swarm into n neighbors and each glowworm i selects a neighbor j with a probability P_{ij} and moves toward it within its decision domains range $R_d(0 < R_d^i < R_s)$, where R_s is a circular sensor range of glowworm i . The position of glowworm i x_i ($x_i \in R^m$, i=1,2,…,n), which is a potential solution. Put x_i into the objective function and gain the fitness function value $J(x_i)$ and luciferin value l_i. Estimate the solution with luciferin value. The algorithm can gain the optimal value of functions. The equations that modeled the luciferin-update, probability distribution used to select a neighbor, movement update and local-decision range update are given below Equation 4.11:

$$l_i(t) = \max\{(0, (1-\rho)*l_i(t-1)+\Upsilon*J(x_i(t)))\} \quad (4.11)$$

$$P_j(t) = \frac{l_j(t)}{\sum_{k \in N_l(t)} l_k(t)} \quad (4.12)$$

$$x_i(t+1) = x_i(t) + s\left(\frac{x_j(t)-x_i(t)}{\|x_j(t)-x_i(t)\|}\right) \quad (4.13)$$

$$r_d^i(t+1) = \frac{r_s}{1+\beta * D_i(t)} \quad (4.14)$$

where

$$N_i(t) = \{j: \|x_j(t) - x_i(t)\| < r_d^i(t); l_i(t) < l_j(t)\} \quad (4.15)$$

is neighbors of glowworm consisting of those glowworms that have a relatively higher luciferin value and that are located within a dynamic decision domain. If the luciferin value of glowworm i is greater than j's and the distance between the glowworm i and j is less than the dynamic decision domain, divide glowworm j into the neighbors of glowworm i . where

$$D_i(t) = \frac{N_i(t)}{\pi * r_s^2} \quad (4.16)$$

is the neighbor-density of glowworm *i* at iteration *t* and β is a constant parameter. The constant parameter β affects the rate of change of the neighborhood range. The constant parameter ρ decides whether algorithm has memory. A value ρ = 0 renders the algorithm memory less where the luciferin value of each glowworm depends only on the fitness value of its current position. However, ρ (∈0 , 1] leads to the reflection of the cumulative goodness of the path followed by the glowworms in their current luciferin values. The constant parameter γ can scale the function fitness values. The value of step-size *s* influences the range of objective function.

4.7. OPITMAL HEART DISEASE PREDICTION USING FUZZY SUPPORT VECTOR MACHINE

To resolve unclassifiable regions, here fuzzy membership functions while realizing the same classification results for the data of heart disease prediction system. To do this, for class i we define one-dimensional membership functions m_{ij} (x) on the directions orthogonal to the optimal separating hyper planes D_j (x) = 0 as follows;

1. For i = j

$$m_{ij}(x) = \begin{cases} 1 & \text{for } D_i(x) > 1 \\ D_i(X) & \text{otherwise} \end{cases} \quad (4.17)$$

2. For $i \neq j$

$$m_{ij}(x) = \begin{cases} 1 & \text{for } D_j(x) < -1 \\ -D_j(x) & \text{otherwise} \end{cases} \quad (4.18)$$

There is only training data set i is available where it is assumed as $D_i > 1$ to take all classes as 1 initially. Else it is assigned with $D_i(x)$ data value.

4.8. RESULTS AND DISCUSSION

The experiments are conducted in the matlab simulation environment where the performance evaluation between the proposed method namely Heart disease prediction using Alpha Rough Set Theory combined with Fuzzy SVM (ARST-FSVM) with our previous work Fuzzy Rough Set Theory combined with Support Vector Machine (FRS - SVM) and the existing methods namely Coronary Heart Disease prediction using Particle Swarm Optimization Approach (CHD-PSO), Artificial Neural Network based Prediction (ANN) is done. The performance metrics that are considered in this research work for the comparison evaluation are, "Accuracy, Precision, Recall, F-Measure". The performance evaluation are shown and explained in the following sub sections.

4.8.1. Accuracy Comparison

Accuracy is defined as the proportion of true positives and true negatives among the total number of results obtained. Accuracy is evaluated as,

$$\text{Accuracy} = \frac{(\text{True positive} + \text{True negative})}{(\text{True positive} + \text{True negative} + \text{False positive} + \text{False negative})} \quad (4.19)$$

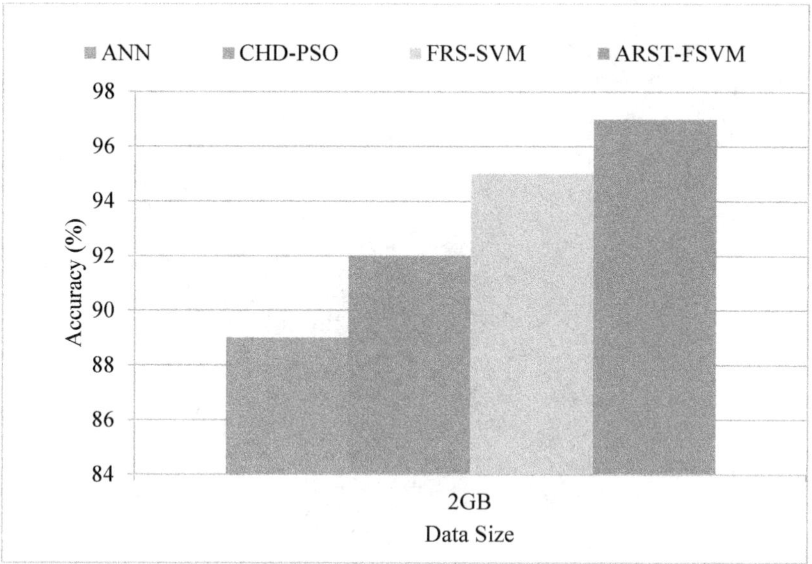

Figure 4.1. Comparison evaluation of Accuracy

From the above graph mentioned in (Figure-4.1), it is proved that the proposed method namely ARST-FSVM can provide better performance result than the existing research methodologies. From the analytical evaluation of the results, it can be proved that the proposed methodology ARST-FSVM shows 2% better performance than FRS_SVM, 5% better than CHD-PSO, 9% better performance than ANN method.

4.8.2. Precision Comparison

Precision value is evaluated according to the relevant information at true positive prediction, false positive.

$$\text{Precision} = \frac{\text{True Positive}}{(\text{True Positive} + \text{False Positive})} \tag{4.20}$$

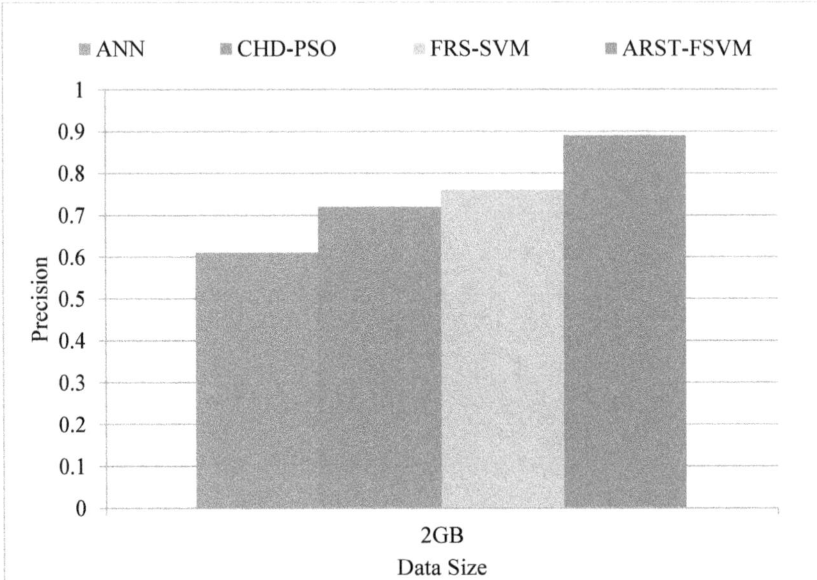

Figure 4.2. Comparison evaluation of Precision

From the above graph it is proved that the proposed method namely ARST-FSVM can provide better performance result than the existing research methodologies in terms of precision. From the analytical evaluation of the results, it can be proved that the proposed methodology ARST-FSVM shows 17% better outcome than FRS-SVM, 24% better than CHD-PSO, 46% better performance than ANN method.

4.8.3. Comparison of Recall

Recall value is evaluated according to the retrieval of information at true positive prediction, false negative.

$$\text{Recall} = \frac{\text{True Positive}}{(\text{True positive} + \text{False negative})} \quad (4.21)$$

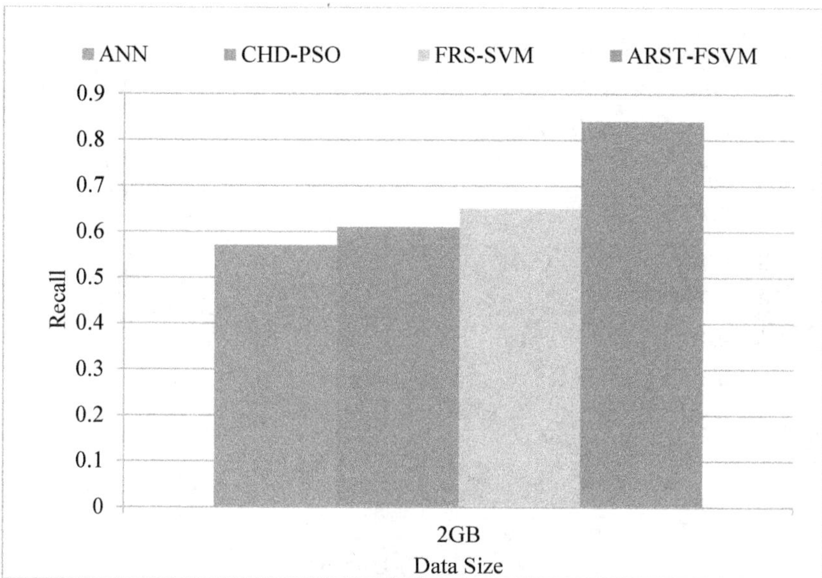

Figure 4.3. Comparison evaluation of Recall

From the above graph it is proved that the proposed method namely ARST-FSVM can provide better performance result than the existing research methodologies. From the analytical evaluation of the results, it can be proved that the proposed methodology ARST-FSVM shows 29 % better result than FRS-SVM, 38% better performance than CHD-PSO, 47% better performance than ANN method

4.8.4. Comparison of F-Measure

The F-Measure computes some average of the information retrieval precision and recall metrics

$$\mathrm{F-Measure} = \frac{2 * \mathrm{precision.recall}}{\mathrm{precision} + \mathrm{recall}} \tag{4.22}$$

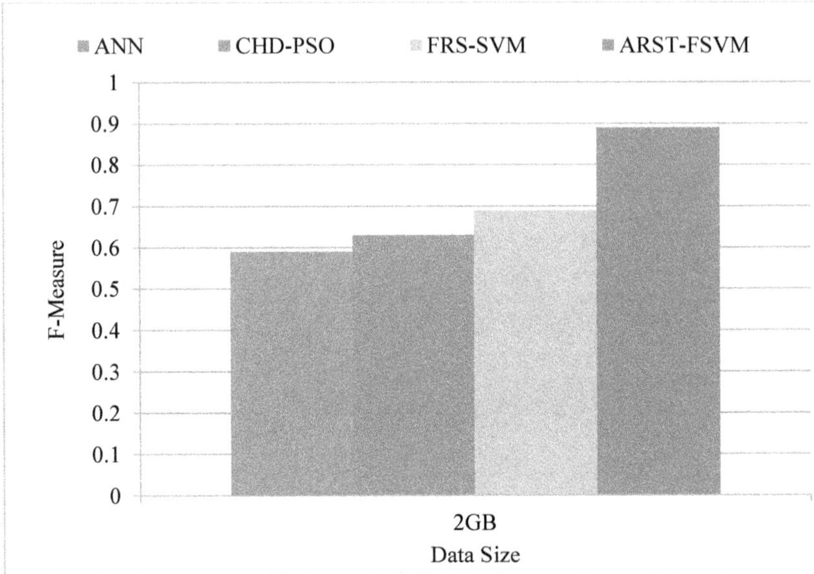

Figure 4.4. Comparison evaluation of F-measure

From the above graph it is proved that the proposed method namely ARST-FSVM can provide better performance result than the existing research methodologies. From the analytical evaluation of the results, it can be proved that the proposed methodology ARST-FSVM shows 29% better outcome than FRS-SVM, 41% better than CHD-PSO, 51% better performance than ANN method.

4.9. SUMMARY

Heart disease prediction process is the most concerned research issue which is focused in this research method by introducing the framework namely Heart disease prediction using Alpha Rough Set Theory combined with Fuzzy SVM (ARST-FSVM). In this research method, Modified K-Means clustering algorithm is used for preprocessing the input dataset which would avoid the noisy data present in the database. Then missing data value in the database is handled using normalization technique where NLLS imputation is applied. And then feature dimensionality reduction is done using Alpha rough set theory (α-RST) approach. From those reduced feature set, optimal feature selection in terms of relevancy is done using Hybrid Bee colony algorithm with Glowworm Swarm Optimization (HBC-GSO) approach. Finally heart disease prediction is done using classifier namely fuzzy based SVM. The overall research method ensures that the proposed research technique leads to ensure it can lead to optimal and accurate heart disease diagnosis outcome.

CHAPTER 5

A RELIABLE AND ACCURATE HEART DISEASE PREDICTION SYSTEM

Heart disease is the most common found risk factor which causes more peoples in the dangerous way with the more threatening issues. Careless treatment provided to the heart disease might cause death which should identify correctly and has to be well handled. In our previous research methods heart disease diagnosis is performed by using different data mining techniques. However those methods fail to provide the optimal outcome in case of more missing value information in the dataset which is larger in size. These problems are focused and resolved in the proposed research method by introducing the Accurate and reliable heart disease prediction with the concern of Risk factors using Hybrid Rough Set-Hybrid Multi Class SVM (HRS-HMCSVM). The proposed research method can optimally predict the heart disease occurrence earlier with increased prediction accuracy. In this research method Hybrid K-Means clustering algorithm is applied to preprocess the dataset. After preprocessing, missing value replacement is done by using imputation methods. And then dimensionality reduction is done by using Hybrid Rough set theory concept which is sent to feature selection module where the optimal features are extracted by using Hybrid Improved Bee Colony with Cuckoo Search Algorithm. Finally, Classification of the dataset is done using Fuzzy SVM approach.

5.1. INTRODUCTION

Recently, health problems are seen increased in alarming heights every day owing to the modern life style, genetic reasons, food habits, stress etc. (Babaoglu et al., 2010). Particularly, heart disease has emerged to be more widely seen in the recent times, which, in turn, indicates that there is a huge risk for human life of people. Every individual has multiple values for Blood Pressure (BP), cholesterol and Pulse Rate (PR).But based on medically established results, the normal values of BP is 120/90, cholesterol is and pulse rate is 72. As per World Health Organization (WHO) report, CardioVascular Diseases (CVDs) would be the largest cause of death and disability in India by 2020 (Chandra and Deekshatulu, 2012).

Heart disease is the huge threat affecting the world. Like the earlier scourge-bubonic plague, yellow fever, and smallpox; Cardiovascular Disease (CVD) not just hits a considerable portion of the population with no warning but leads to extended agony and disability in a greater count (Chen et al., 2010). Luckily, research efforts aimed at the cause, diagnosis, treatment, and prevention of heart disease is speeding up with a quicker pace. Specifically, the past few decades has noticed a break-through expansion for getting to know about the structure and functioning of the cardiovascular system, sometimes through methods requiring to penetrating into the skin and also, with an increase in accuracy, through non-invasive techniques (Chi et al., 2010).

Usually, data mining is described as the procedure of evaluating the data from a variety of perspectives and then providing its summary in the form of resourceful information, which can be exploited for increasing the revenue, reduce expenses, or both (Han et al., 2011). Data mining software is one among several analytical tools employed for data analysis. It lets the users to evaluate the data from diverse dimensions or angles, classify it, and then the result is a summary of the identified associations (Data et al., 2010). In technical terms, data mining can be considered to be the process of figuring out the correlations or patterns among numerous fields in huge relational databases.

The prediction of the heart disease can be carried out by employing predictive data mining (Phyu, 2009). The description regarding the predictive data mining is provided in the section below. The heart disease prediction can be done in data mining strategy. There are two essential steps that are needed for the prediction of the heart disease. The first one refers to the diagnosis of heart disease and then the treatment in accordance with the diagnosis process for the heart disease taken in concern.

The heart disease diagnosis starts with getting a medical history of the patient to identify if he has been affected with the disease earlier. Risk factors have to be evaluated, and then testing may be necessary to confirm the heart disease. The health care provider will attempt to select the testing modality, which will best offer the diagnosis, and in case heart disease exists, the presence of any impairment, if any, has to be determined.

In this research method, earlier prediction of heart disease is done with increased prediction accuracy. In this research method Hybrid K-Means clustering algorithm is applied to preprocess the dataset. After preprocessing, Missing value replacement is done by using imputation methods. And then dimensionality reduction is done by using Hybrid Rough set theory concept which is sent to feature selection module where the optimal features are extracted by using Hybrid Improved Bee Colony with Cuckoo Search Algorithm. Finally, Classification of the dataset is done using Fuzzy SVM approach.

5.2. RELIABLE AND ACCURATE HEART DISEASE PREDICTION SYSTEM

From huge datasets, hidden patterns were acquired with the help of the data mining concept, which is developed as a research field. As like data mining concept, medical science has also been come out with huge hope, and it generates data from the clinical report and from patient's symptoms record. So, in medical science also, data mining conceit is utilized for gather the data. The acquired hidden patterns were utilized for clinical diagnosis. Nevertheless, medical datasets were wide spread and these data has to be arranged and combined with the hospital management systems.

These problems are focused and resolved in the proposed research method by introducing the Accurate and reliable heart disease prediction with the concern of Risk factors using Hybrid Rough Set-Hybrid Multi Class SVM (HRS-HMCSVM).

The proposed research method can optimally predict the heart disease occurrence earlier with increased prediction accuracy. In this research method

- Hybrid K-Means clustering algorithm for preprocessing
- Missing value replacement using imputation methods
- Dimensionality reduction using Hybrid Rough set theory concept
- Hybrid Improved Bee Colony with Cuckoo Search Algorithm for optimal feature selection
- Classification of the dataset using Fuzzy SVM approach

The detailed explanation of the proposed research technique is given in the following sub sections.

5.3. HYBRID K-MEANS CLUSTERING ALGORITHM FOR PREPROCESSING

This clustering algorithm is used for performing preprocessing by utilizing similarity calculation procedure. This method can ensure the efficient preprocessing on data set by removing unwanted outliers from the present dataset. Here optimal initial centroid selection is introduced newly in this method which is done based relevancy factor. More irrelevant features would be taken centroids based on which grouping would be done and remaining features that done represent any group would be omitted as outlier.

Hybrid K-means is introduced to optimally selecting the initial centroids by integrating it with the ant colony algorithm which is novel research in this method. One advantage of ant clustering algorithm is, without any information about classification, this algorithm can finish a primary clustering. However two problems exist. One is, when the algorithm ends up, there are some data not to be assigned to a stack. We call them free data, including the data ants loaded and the data located on the grid individually.

Another problem is, if data is placed in a data stack incorrectly, it will cost long time to be moved to the correct data stack by ant. K-means algorithm can make the square error of k clustering minimize. In case of many data, it is effective and smart. However you must assign k value before clustering. It is difficult to some inexperienced users. On the other hand, the choosing of initial clustering centers will make influence on the final clustering result.

5.3.1. Ant Clustering Algorithm

Ant colony algorithm is a novel optimization method by simulating evolution. Ant clustering algorithm is its branch, which is a kind of clustering algorithm based on swarm intelligence and is often applied in image segmentation. Researchers observed the fact that ants can classify their ant babies automatically and orderly. Researchers were enlightened from this, ant clustering algorithm was proposed. Its basic idea is that all un clustering objects are put on a two-dimensional grid. Each object takes an initial place randomly. Ants are also on the grid and can move randomly. When an ant runs into an object, it will measure colony similarity within its local range. This data will be transformed into the probability that the ant moves the object by. The ant will pick up or drop the object according to the value of this probability. The transportation of objects by ants is a process of self organization clustering. In the end, different clusters on the flat will take shape.

Definitions of colony similarity: Colony similarity is the similarity between an un-clustering object and other objects within its local range. The expression of that is given Equation 5.1

$$f(O_i) = \begin{cases} \frac{1}{\pi r^2} \sum_{o_j \in Neigh(r)} \left(1 - \frac{d(o_i - o_j)}{\alpha}\right) \\ 0 \qquad\qquad \text{otherwise} \end{cases} \tag{5.1}$$

Here: Neigh(r) denotes ant's local range. It refers to a circular area that r is its radius on the grid. $d(o_i, o_j)$ presents the distance between object O_i and O_j in the attribute space. Euclidean distance and cosine distance are often used to express the distance between objects. α is defined as a co-efficient of colony similarity.

Probability transformation function: The task of probability transformation function is to transform colony similarity into the probability of ants transporting un-clustering object. Colony similarity is its variable. The co-domain of probability transformation function is from 0 to 1. It usually can be drawn into two corresponding curves on the co-ordinate. One expresses the probability of pick-up, another expresses the probability of drop. The regulation of probability transformation function is as followed: The more the colony similarity is, the less the probability of pick-up is; the less the colony similarity is, the more the probability of pick-up is. To the probability of drop, visa versa. According to this principle, we can choose sigmoid function as probability transformation function. The probability of pick-up and the probability of drop are individually defined as followed in Equation 5.2 and 5.3:

$$P_p = 1 - \text{Sigmoid}\ (f(O_i)) \tag{5.2}$$

$$P_d = \text{Sigmoid}\ (f(O_i)) \tag{5.3.}$$

Here: $\text{Sigmoid}\ (x) = \frac{1-e^{-\alpha}}{1+e^{-\alpha}}$

c is a constant. The more it is, the faster convergence of algorithm is.

5.3.2. K Means Algorithm

K-means algorithm is an algorithm based on partition, the algorithm assumes that there is a database consisting of n objects and k is known as the number of clustering. We can make use of the partition method to build k partitions ($k \leq n$). Each partition denotes a cluster. Clustering is also based on the similarity between objects. Usually the distance such as Euclidean distance and cosine distance is measured as the similarity. The result of clustering analysis is that objects in the same class are as similar as possible and objects belonging to different classes are as un-similar as possible. The often used partition-methods are k-means algorithm and k-center algorithm.

K objects are randomly chosen from n objects as initial clustering centers. Then the algorithm calculates the distance from each object to k clustering centers and judge which distance is nearest to the clustering center. If one object is that, it will be assigned to this cluster. When all the work of computation is done, it will form k new clusters. Next, the algorithm re-computes a mean value of each new cluster as its new clustering center. According to above procedure, the algorithm will repeat calculating the distance and iterating till criterion function converges. The sum of square error is often-used as the criterion function. It's defined as in Equation 5.4:

$$E = \sum_{i=1}^{k} \sum_{p \in C_i} |p - m_i|^2 \tag{5.4}$$

E is the sum of square error to all objects in the database. P is a point in the space that expresses a given object. m_i is the mean of clustering C_i. According to this criterion, data belonging to the same class is as more similar as possible and data from different classes are as more different as possible.

5.3.3. Hybrid Clustering Algorithm

One advantage of ant clustering algorithm is, without any information about classification, this algorithm can finish a primary clustering. However two problems exist. One is, when the algorithm ends up, there are some data not to be assigned to a stack. We call them free data, including the data ants loaded and the data located on the grid individually. Another problem is, if data is placed in a data stack incorrectly, it will cost long time to be moved to the correct data stack by ant. K-means algorithm can make the square error of k clustering minimize. In case of many data, it is effective and smart. However you must assign k value before clustering. It is difficult to some inexperienced users. On the other hand, the choosing of initial clustering centers will make influence on the final clustering result.

Hybrid clustering algorithm is based on the combination of ant clustering algorithm and K-means algorithm. According to random ergodic theory, ant clustering algorithm doesn't need priori knowledge to do clustering analysis. This algorithm can avoid local optimization but will cost long time to compute. K-means algorithm needs an initial clustering to analyze by means of certainty inspiring principle. However it can converge fast. Two algorithms have complementary advantages. K-means algorithm is convergent in theory. K-means algorithm is able to remove the incorrect point quickly and assign free data object to the corresponding cluster. Hybrid algorithm doesn't need input initial cluster information and can avoid bad results because of incorrect initial information. Obviously, the combination will accelerate the running of algorithm and improve clustering. B. The description of hybrid clustering algorithm Hybrid clustering algorithm is described as following:

a) Each data object is made to do clustering with ant clustering algorithm.

b) From a, k clusters and their clustering centers are chosen.

c) Input above-information and cluster with K-means algorithm.

d) Output the result.

5.4. MISSING VALUE REPLACEMENT USING IMPUTATION METHODS

Incomplete datasets can lead to misleading conclusions, as demonstrated by Kidson and Trenberth (1988), who assessed the impact of missing data on general circulation statistics by systematically decreasing the amount of available training data. They determined that the ratio of the Root Mean Square Error (RMSE) in the monthly mean to the daily standard deviation was two to three times higher when the missing data was spaced randomly compared to space equally, and RMSE increased by up to a factor of two when the missing data occurred in one block. Therefore, the spacing of the missing data can have an impact on statistical analyses. It is useful to consider how to best replace, or impute, the missing data.

In this research work Full Information Maximum Likelihood method is utilized for replacing the missing value information accurately. In this method, missing values are not replaced or imputed, but the missing data is handled within the analysis model. The model is estimated by a full information maximum likelihood method, that way all available information is used to estimate the model. In full information maximum likelihood the population parameters are estimated that would most likely produce the estimates from the sample data that is analyzed.

Examples of models that are often estimated by full information maximum likelihood are structural equation models and multi-level models or growth models. Multiple imputation and full information maximum likelihood will come to similar results when outcome data are missing and the same information is incorporated in a multiple imputation model as in full information maximum likelihood estimation [3].

Probably the most pragmatic missing data estimation approach for structural equation modeling is Full Information Maximum Likelihood (FIML), which has been shown to produce unbiased parameter estimates and standard errors under MAR and MCAR. FIML, sometimes called “direct maximum likelihood,” "raw maximum likelihood" or just "ML," is currently available in all major SEM packages. FIML requires that missing values to be at least MAR (i.e., either MAR or MCAR are ok). The process works by estimating a likelihood function for each individual based on the variables that are present so that all the available data are used. For example, there may be some variables with data for all 389 cases but some variables may have data for only 320 of the cases. Model fit information in is derived from a summation across fit functions for individual cases, and, thus, model fit information is based on all 389 cases. Rather than the traditional approach to calculating chi-square, FIML estimates two models, the H0 model and the H1 model.

The H0 model is the "unrestricted" model, meaning that all variables are correlated. The H1 model is the specified model. The difference between the two log-likelihoods is used to derive the chi-square. This approach allows one to use all the available information in the variables. There is good evidence to suggest that using modern missing data estimation approaches may be reasonable even if missingness is non ignorable (i.e., MAR assumptions have not been met) provided correlates of missingness (auxiliary variables) are included in the model. Inclusion of auxiliary variables has the most impact when their association with missingness is high (e.g., > .4) and when the amount of missing data is large. Graham shows that two methods of modeling these auxiliary variables (either as dependent variables or correlated variables) are equally effective in reducing parameter biases, but including auxiliary variables as correlates has a greater impact on reducing biases in model fit.

Suppose that y = (y1, y2,...yp)' has a multivariate normal distribution with mean μ and covariance matrix $\sum$ and that $y_1, y_2, \ldots, y_n$ is a random sample of the vector y. Specific elements of the vectors y_k, k=1,2,..n may be unobserved so that the data set comprising of n rows (the different cases) and p columns (variable 1,2,...,p) have missing values. Let y_k denote a vector with incomplete observations, then this vector can be replaces by $y_k^* = X_k y_k$ where Xk is a selection matrix and yk has typical elements ($y_{k1}, y_{k2}, \ldots y_{kp}$) with one or more of the y_{kj}^s missing, j=1,2,...p. For example suppose p=3 and that variable 2 is unobserved then it is given as like in Equation 5.5

$$y_k^* = \begin{bmatrix} y_{k1} \\ y_{k2} \end{bmatrix} = \begin{bmatrix} 1 & 0 & 0 \\ 0 & 0 & 1 \end{bmatrix} \begin{bmatrix} y_{k1} \\ y_{k2} \\ y_{k3} \end{bmatrix} \tag{5.5}$$

From the above example it can easily be seen that X_k is based on an identity matrix with rows deleted according to missing elements of y_k. If an observed vector y_k contains no unobserved values, then X_k is equal to the identity matrix and hence $y_k^* = yk$. Without loss in generality, (y_1, y_2,.. y_n) can be replaced with $(y_1^*, y_2^*, \ldots y_n^*)$ where y_k^*, k=1,2,...n has a normal distribution with mean $X_k\mu$ and covariance matrix $X_k \sum X'_k$. The log likelihood for the non missing data is $\sum_{k=1}^{n} log\, f(y_k^*, \mu_k, \sum_k)$.

5.5. DIMENSIONALITY REDUCTION USING HYBRID ROUGH SET THEORY CONCEPT

Here dimensionality reduction is achieved by integrating rough set concept with the learning algorithms that can ensure the accurate dimensionality reduction. Artificial neural network for accurately find the objects to be added in the set.

1) The framework of hybridizing RST and ANN based set all weights of units to random values ranging from -1.0 to +1.0.
2) Set an input pattern to the neurons of the net's input layer.
3) Activate each neuron of the following layer.

These two techniques can be used for both classification and regression tasks without any converting mechanism. Incorporating these two technologies in one as an Intelligent Rough Neural Network System for efficient processing of medical data base is described in this section. The proposed hybrid system uses RST for preprocessing of data and ANN for classification or prediction. Some researchers have proposed and used similar integrated method in other applications.

Algorithm: IRNNS

Given: Medical data set.

Objective: Obtain crisp set of influential parameters and construct suitable ANN architecture for prediction.

// Pre-processing phase using RST.//

Step 1. Discretize the data.

Step 2. Construct the information system.

Step 3. Select influential parameters in the form of reduct set by applying Reduct algorithm.

Step 4. Check the selected parameters by considering biological importance. If satisfied go to Step 5 for training ANN else go to Step 1.

// ANN construction and training phase.//

Step 5. Data set (n_i, n_t) n = 1,2, … k, where input in and target tn. Split the data into three subsets as training, cross-validation and test sets.

Step 6. Construct suitable ANN architecture. Structuring ANN with supervised back propagation learning algorithm includes following steps:

1) Set all weights of units to random values ranging from -1.0 to +1.0.

2) Set an input pattern to the neurons of the net's input layer.

3) Activate each neuron of the following layer.

(Multiply the weight values of the connections leading to the neuron with the output values of the proceeding neurons and add up these values. Pass the result to an activation function, which computing the output value of this neuron.)

4) Repeat this until the output layer is reached.

5) Compare the calculated output pattern to the desired target pattern and compute an error value.

6) Change all weights of each weight matrix using the formula Weight (old) + learning rate * output error * output (neurons i) * output (neurons i+1) * (1 - output (neurons i+1))

7) Go to Step 2.

8) The algorithm ends, if all output patterns match their target patterns.

Step 7. Now, the constructed ANN is ready for prediction or classification. (The performance of this network was subsequently optimized by varying the number of nodes in the hidden layer and remove redundant nodes.)

5.6. HYBRID IMPROVED BEE COLONY WITH CUCKOO SEARCH ALGORITHM FOR OPTIMAL FEATURE SELECTION

Here Hybrid improved bee colony and cuckoo search is introduced for the optimal feature selection which can achieve the reduced convergence time. Artificial bee colony algorithm and Cuckoo search algorithm all belong to swarm intelligence heuristics. Artificial bee colony algorithm has relatively high convergence rate, but it is easy to fall into local optimum. Cuckoo search algorithm not only has the general characteristics of intelligent algorithm, but also has the rapid global convergence which genetic algorithm and particle swarm optimization can't be compared with. And at the same time, it can effectively escape from local optimum. But it also has problems such as the performance limits to convergence speed caused by the lack of information sharing mechanism among individuals in the population. This paper puts forward the improvements of artificial bee colony's population update strategy. It is found that the Lévy flight search strategy of Cuckoo search algorithm is a kind of global search operator and can escape from local optimum. And the inferior individual's elimination mechanism can improve population quality advantages. At the same time, artificial bee colony algorithm's effective information sharing mechanism makes up the defects of Cuckoo search algorithm to some extent. This work introduces Lévy flight search strategy into update operations to the food source's location of mixed artificial bee colony algorithm to enhance the global search capability of artificial bee colony algorithm, taking full advantage of the random walk characteristic of Lévy flight to have huge leap and several changes in direction, thus it can effectively prevent colony from being bound by local attractors and expand search space. The improved update mode to food sources is as Equation (5.6):

$$x_i^j(t+1) = x_i^j(t) + L(\lambda) \otimes \left(x_i^j(t) - x_{best}^j\right), 1 < \lambda \leq 3 \qquad (5.6)$$

In the formula, x_{best}^j is the location of the current best food source in the colony; $L(\lambda)$ is the hop path of random search whose step size obeys Lévy distribution and its length and direction are uncertain; Parameter λ is scale parameter and $\lambda = 1 + \beta$; $\otimes$ is the vector operator. The implementation process of mixed artificial bee colony algorithm is as follows:

(1) Set the initial parameters, including the number of colonies N, the colony's maximum evolution generation, the maximum number of iterations and colony's group information;

(2) Randomly initialize the bee colony (food source) $X_0(N)$, and calculate fitness values of individuals in population.

(3) Circulate (when the loop condition is satisfied) or skip to (9);

(4) Employed foragers conduct a global search to generate new locations according to formula (9), and select relatively good candidates for solutions of the next generation according to the merit-based selection mechanism.

(5) Eliminate or reserve the colony according to selection strategy: calculate the probability of being selected according to following equation 5.7 & 5.8

$$P_i = \frac{fit_i}{\sum_{n=1}^{N} fit_j} \tag{5.7}$$

$$fit_i = \begin{cases} \dfrac{1}{1+f_i} & f_i \geq 0 \\ 1 + abs(f_i) & f_i < 0 \end{cases} \tag{5.8}$$

(6) Onlookers select the locations of food sources according to p_i, update the locations of food sources according to formula (9) and select relatively good candidates for solutions of the next generation according to the greedy principle;

(7) Scouts re-initialized to generate new solutions.

(8) Calculate and record the optimum solution of the current colony and then return to step (3);

(9) End.

5.7. CLASSIFICATION OF THE DATASET USING FUZZY SVM APPROACH

To resolve unclassifiable regions, here fuzzy membership functions while realizing the same classification results for the data of heart disease prediction system. To do this, for class i we define one-dimensional membership functions m_{ij} (x) on the directions orthogonal to the optimal separating hyper planes D_j (x) = 0 as follows;

1. For i = j

$$M_{ij}(x) = \begin{cases} 1 & \text{for } D_i(x) > 1 \\ D_i(X) & \text{otherwise} \end{cases} \tag{5.9}$$

2. For i ≠ j

$$M_{ij}(x) = \begin{cases} 1 & \text{for } D_j(x) < -1 \\ -D_j(x) & \text{otherwise} \end{cases} \tag{5.10}$$

There is only training data set i is available where it is assumed as $D_i > 1$ to take all classes as 1 initially. Else it is assigned with $D_i(x)$ data value.

5.8. RESULTS AND DISCUSSION

The experiments are conducted in the matlab simulation environment where the performance evaluation between the proposed method namely Heart disease prediction using HRS-HMCSVM with our previous work Alpha Rough Set Theory combined with Fuzzy SVM (ARST-FSVM), Fuzzy Rough Set Theory combined with Support Vector Machine (FRS - SVM) and the existing methods namely Coronary Heart Disease prediction using Particle Swarm Optimization Approach (CHD-PSO), Artificial Neural Network based Prediction (ANN) is done.

The performance metrics that are considered in this research work for the comparison evaluation are, "Accuracy, Precision, Recall, F-Measure". The performance evaluation are shown and explained in the following sub sections.

5.8.1. Numerical Analysis of Accuracy

Accuracy is defined as the proportion of true positives and true negatives among the total number of results obtained. Accuracy is evaluated as,

$$\text{Accuracy} = \frac{(\text{True positive} + \text{True negative})}{(\text{True positive} + \text{True negative} + \text{False positive} + \text{False negative})} \tag{5.11}$$

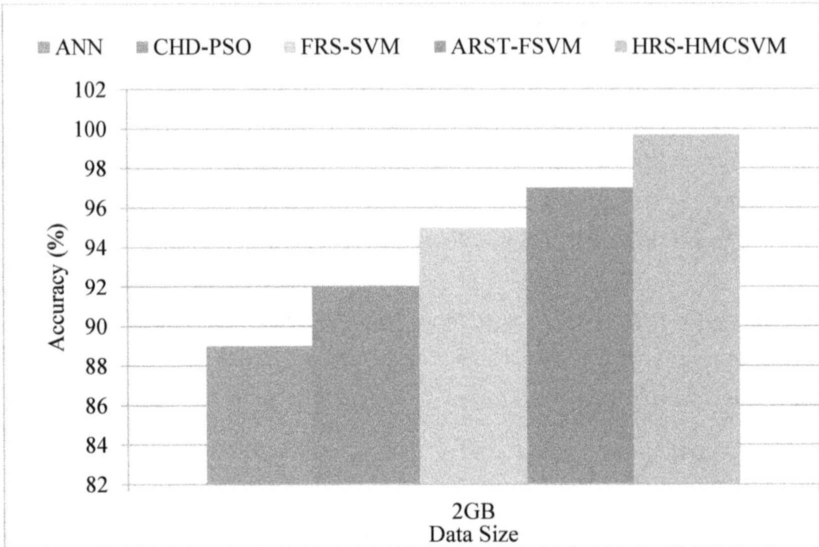

Figure 5.1. Simulation outcome of Accuracy

From the above graph mentioned in (Figure-5.1), it is proved that the proposed method namely HRS-HMCSVM can provide better performance result than the existing research methodologies. From the analytical evaluation of the results, it can be proved that the proposed methodology HRS-HMCSVM is 3% better than ARST-FSVM, 5% better performance than FRS_SVM, 8% better than CHD-PSO, 12% better performance than ANN method.

5.8.2. Numerical Analysis of Precision

Precision value is evaluated according to the relevant information at true positive prediction, false positive.

$$\text{Precision} = \frac{\text{True Positive}}{(\text{True Positive} + \text{False Positive})} \tag{5.12}$$

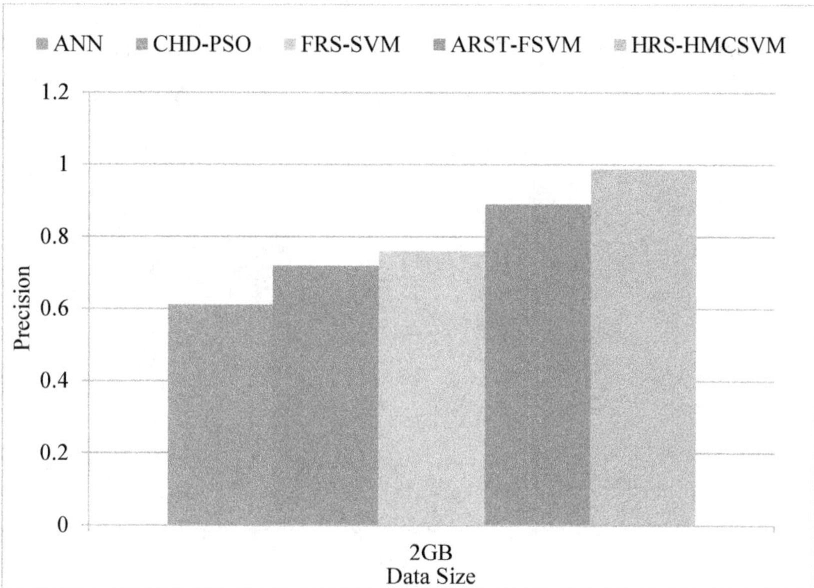

Figure 5.2. Simulation outcome of Precision

From the above graph it is proved that the proposed method namely HRS-HMCSVM can provide better performance result than the existing research methodologies in terms of precision. From the analytical evaluation of the results, it can be proved that the proposed methodology HRS-HMCSVM is 11% better than ARST-FSVM, 30% better outcome than FRS-SVM, 37% better than CHD-PSO, 32% better performance than ANN method.

5.8.3. Numerical Analysis of Recall

Recall value is evaluated according to the retrieval of information at true positive prediction, false negative.

$$\text{Recall} = \frac{\text{True Positive}}{(\text{True positive} + \text{False negative})} \tag{5.13}$$

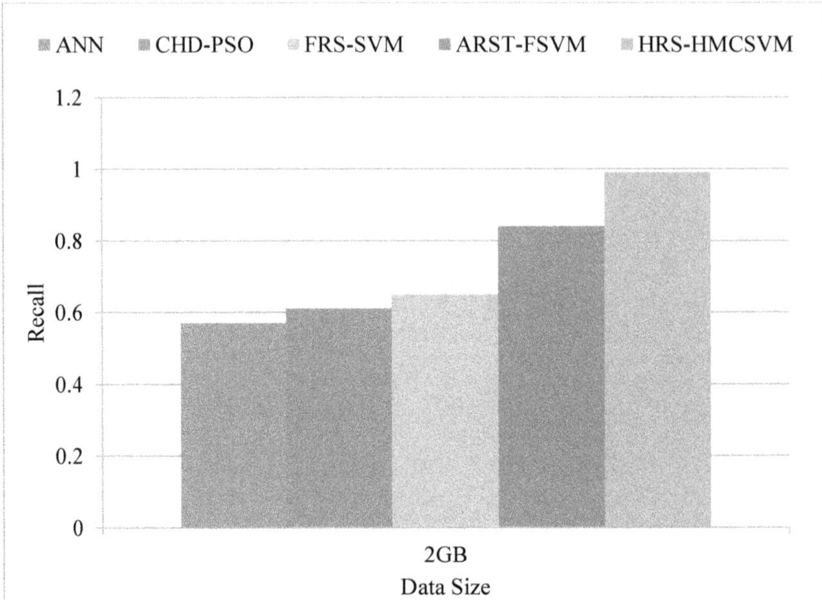

Figure 5.3. Simulation outcome of Recall

From the above graph it is proved that the proposed method namely HRS-HMCSVM can provide better performance result than the existing research methodologies. From the analytical evaluation of the results, it can be proved that the proposed methodology HRS-HMCSVM is 18% better than ARST-FSVM, 52% better result than FRS-SVM, 62% better performance than CHD-PSO, 74% better performance than ANN method

5.8.4. Numerical Analysis of F-Measure

The F-Measure computes some average of the information retrieval precision and recall metrics

$$\mathrm{F-Measure} = \frac{2 * \mathrm{precision.recall}}{\mathrm{precision + recall}} \tag{5.14}$$

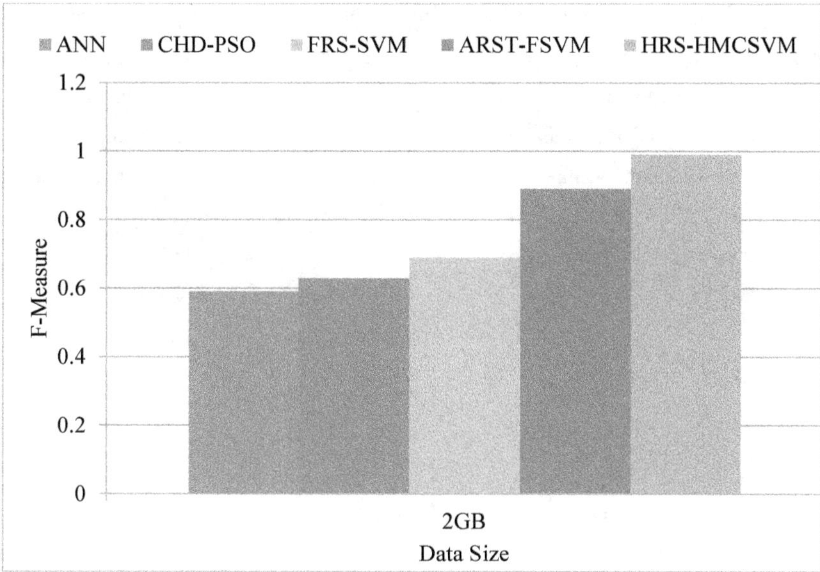

Figure 5.4. Simulation outcome of F-measure

From the above graph it is proved that the proposed method namely HRS-HMCSVM can provide better performance result than the existing research methodologies. From the analytical evaluation of the results, it can be proved that the proposed methodology HRS-HMCSVM is 11% better than ARST-FSVM, 43 % better outcome than FRS-SVM, 57% better than CHD-PSO, 68% better performance than ANN method.

5.9. SUMMARY

Heart disease has increased quickly by reason of varying lifestyle combined with improper or lack of physical exercise, foretelling and averting the heart diseases at prior stage has turn out to be a significant action as in every year root to death. Plentiful researchers presented in the current work for health disease prediction. These problems are focused and resolved in the proposed research method by introducing the Accurate and reliable heart disease prediction with the concern of Risk factors using Hybrid Rough Set-Hybrid Multi Class SVM (HRS-HMCSVM). The proposed research method can optimally predict the heart disease occurrence earlier with increased prediction accuracy. In this research method Hybrid K-Means clustering algorithm is applied to preprocess the dataset. After preprocessing, missing value replacement is done by using imputation methods. And then dimensionality reduction is done by using Hybrid Rough set theory concept which is sent to feature selection module where the optimal features are extracted by using Hybrid Improved Bee Colony with Cuckoo Search Algorithm. Finally, Classification of the dataset is done using Fuzzy SVM approach.

CHAPTER 6

RESULTS AND DISCUSSION

In this research, proposed method has been implemented and evaluated in the mat lab simulation environment. The proposed system is implemented using MATLAB 2014b and the experimentation is performed with i5 processor of 3GB RAM.

6.1. SOFTWARE DESCRIPTION

MATLAB, short for MATrix LABoratory is a programming package specifically designed for quick and easy scientific calculations and I/O. It has literally hundreds of built-in functions for a wide variety of computations and many toolboxes designed for specific research disciplines, including statistics, optimization, solution of partial differential equations, data analysis. Image Processing Toolbox™ provides a comprehensive set of reference-standard algorithms and workflow apps for image processing, analysis, visualization, and algorithm development. You can perform image segmentation, image enhancement, noise reduction, geometric transformations, image registration, and 3D image processing.

Image Processing Toolbox apps let you automate common image processing workflows. You can interactively segment image data, compare image registration techniques, and batch-process large data sets. Visualization functions and apps let you explore images, 3D volumes, and videos; adjust contrast; create histograms; and manipulate regions of interest (ROIs). You can accelerate your algorithms by running them on multi core processors and GPUs. Many toolbox functions support C/C++ code generation for desktop prototyping and embedded vision system deployment.

6.2. DATASET DETAILS

```
1. Title: Heart Disease Databases

2. Source Information:
   (a) Creators:
       -- 1. Hungarian Institute of Cardiology. Budapest: Andras Janosi, M.D.
       -- 2. University Hospital, Zurich, Switzerland: William Steinbrunn, M.D.
       -- 3. University Hospital, Basel, Switzerland: Matthias Pfisterer, M.D.
       -- 4. V.A. Medical Center, Long Beach and Cleveland Clinic Foundation:
             Robert Detrano, M.D., Ph.D.
   (b) Donor: David W. Aha (aha@ics.uci.edu) (714) 856-8779
   (c) Date: July, 1988
```

```
3. Past Usage:
    1. Detrano,~R., Janosi,~A., Steinbrunn,~W., Pfisterer,~M., Schmid,~J.,
       Sandhu,~S., Guppy,~K., Lee,~S., \& Froelicher,~V. (1989).  {\it
       International application of a new probability algorithm for the
       diagnosis of coronary artery disease.}  {\it American Journal of
       Cardiology}, {\it 64},304--310.
       -- International Probability Analysis
       -- Address: Robert Detrano, M.D.
                   Cardiology 111-C
                   V.A. Medical Center
                   5901 E. 7th Street
                   Long Beach, CA 90028
       -- Results in percent accuracy: (for 0.5 probability threshold)
             Data Name:  CDF    CADENZA
          -- Hungarian   77     74
             Long beach  79     77
             Swiss       81     81
          -- Approximately a 77% correct classification accuracy with a
             logistic-regression-derived discriminant function
    2. David W. Aha & Dennis Kibler
       --


          -- Instance-based prediction of heart-disease presence with the
             Cleveland database
             -- NTgrowth: 77.0% accuracy
             --       C4: 74.8% accuracy
    3. John Gennari
       -- Gennari, J.~H., Langley, P, \& Fisher, D. (1989). Models of
          incremental concept formation. {\it Artificial Intelligence, 40},
          11--61.
       -- Results:
          -- The CLASSIT conceptual clustering system achieved a 78.9% accuracy
             on the Cleveland database.

4. Relevant Information:
     This database contains 76 attributes, but all published experiments
     refer to using a subset of 14 of them.  In particular, the Cleveland
     database is the only one that has been used by ML researchers to
     this date.  The "goal" field refers to the presence of heart disease
     in the patient.  It is integer valued from 0 (no presence) to 4.
     Experiments with the Cleveland database have concentrated on simply
     attempting to distinguish presence (values 1,2,3,4) from absence (value
     0).

     The names and social security numbers of the patients were recently
     removed from the database, replaced with dummy values.

     One file has been "processed", that one containing the Cleveland
     database.  All four unprocessed files also exist in this directory.

5. Number of Instances:
        Database:    # of instances:
          Cleveland: 303
          Hungarian: 294
        Switzerland: 123
      Long Beach VA: 200

6. Number of Attributes: 76 (including the predicted attribute)

7. Attribute Information:
   -- Only 14 used
```

```
    -- 1. #3  (age)
    -- 2. #4  (sex)
    -- 3. #9  (cp)
    -- 4. #10 (trestbps)
    -- 5. #12 (chol)
    -- 6. #16 (fbs)
    -- 7. #19 (restecg)
    -- 8. #32 (thalach)
    -- 9. #38 (exang)
    -- 10. #40 (oldpeak)
    -- 11. #41 (slope)
    -- 12. #44 (ca)
    -- 13. #51 (thal)
    -- 14. #58 (num)       (the predicted attribute)

-- Complete attribute documentation:
    1 id: patient identification number
    2 ccf: social security number (I replaced this with a dummy value of 0)
    3 age: age in years
    4 sex: sex (1 = male; 0 = female)
    5 painloc: chest pain location (1 = substernal; 0 = otherwise)
    6 painexer (1 = provoked by exertion; 0 = otherwise)
    7 relrest (1 = relieved after rest; 0 = otherwise)
    8 pncaden (sum of 5, 6, and 7)
    9 cp: chest pain type
      -- Value 1: typical angina
      -- Value 2: atypical angina
      -- Value 3: non-anginal pain
      -- Value 4: asymptomatic
   10 trestbps: resting blood pressure (in mm Hg on admission to the
      hospital)
   11 htn
   12 chol: serum cholestoral in mg/dl
   13 smoke: I believe this is 1 = yes; 0 = no (is or is not a smoker)
   14 cigs (cigarettes per day)
   15 years (number of years as a smoker)
   16 fbs: (fasting blood sugar > 120 mg/dl)  (1 = true; 0 = false)
   17 dm (1 = history of diabetes; 0 = no such history)
   18 famhist: family history of coronary artery disease (1 = yes; 0 = no)
   19 restecg: resting electrocardiographic results
      -- Value 0: normal
      -- Value 1: having ST-T wave abnormality (T wave inversions and/or ST
                  elevation or depression of > 0.05 mV)
      -- Value 2: showing probable or definite left ventricular hypertrophy
                  by Estes' criteria
   20 ekgmo (month of exercise ECG reading)
   21 ekgday(day of exercise ECG reading)
   22 ekgyr (year of exercise ECG reading)
   23 dig (digitalis used furing exercise ECG: 1 = yes; 0 = no)
   24 prop (Beta blocker used during exercise ECG: 1 = yes; 0 = no)
   25 nitr (nitrates used during exercise ECG: 1 = yes; 0 = no)
   26 pro (calcium channel blocker used during exercise ECG: 1 = yes; 0 = no)
   27 diuretic (diuretic used used during exercise ECG: 1 = yes; 0 = no)
   28 proto: exercise protocol
        1 = Bruce
        2 = Kottus
        3 = McHenry
        4 = fast Balke
        5 = Balke
        6 = Noughton
        7 = bike 150 kpa min/min  (Not sure if "kpa min/min" is what was
            written!)
        8 = bike 125 kpa min/min
```

```
     9 = bike 100 kpa min/min
    10 = bike 75 kpa min/min
    11 = bike 50 kpa min/min
    12 = arm ergometer
29 thaldur: duration of exercise test in minutes
30 thaltime: time when ST measure depression was noted
31 met: mets achieved
32 thalach: maximum heart rate achieved
33 thalrest: resting heart rate
34 tpeakbps: peak exercise blood pressure (first of 2 parts)
35 tpeakbpd: peak exercise blood pressure (second of 2 parts)
36 dummy
37 trestbpd: resting blood pressure
38 exang: exercise induced angina (1 = yes; 0 = no)
39 xhypo: (1 = yes; 0 = no)
40 oldpeak = ST depression induced by exercise relative to rest
41 slope: the slope of the peak exercise ST segment
   -- Value 1: upsloping
   -- Value 2: flat
   -- Value 3: downsloping
42 rldv5: height at rest
43 rldv5e: height at peak exercise
44 ca: number of major vessels (0-3) colored by flourosopy
45 restckm: irrelevant
46 exerckm: irrelevant
47 restef: rest raidonuclid (sp?) ejection fraction
48 restwm: rest wall (sp?) motion abnormality
   0 = none
   1 = mild or moderate
   2 = moderate or severe
   3 = akinesis or dyskmem (sp?)
49 exeref: exercise radinalid (sp?) ejection fraction
50 exerwm: exercise wall (sp?) motion
51 thal: 3 = normal; 6 = fixed defect; 7 = reversable defect
52 thalsev: not used
53 thalpul: not used
54 earlobe: not used
55 cmo: month of cardiac cath (sp?)  (perhaps "call")
56 cday: day of cardiac cath (sp?)
57 cyr: year of cardiac cath (sp?)
58 num: diagnosis of heart disease (angiographic disease status)
   -- Value 0: < 50% diameter narrowing
   -- Value 1: > 50% diameter narrowing
   (in any major vessel: attributes 59 through 68 are vessels)
59 lmt
60 ladprox
61 laddist
62 diag
63 cxmain
64 ramus
65 om1
66 om2
67 rcaprox
68 rcadist
69 lvx1: not used
70 lvx2: not used
71 lvx3: not used
72 lvx4: not used
73 lvf: not used
74 cathef: not used
75 junk: not used
76 name: last name of patient
    (I replaced this with the dummy string "name")
```

```
9. Missing Attribute Values: Several.  Distinguished with value -9.0.

10. Class Distribution:
        Database:      0   1   2   3   4 Total
          Cleveland: 164  55  36  35  13   303
          Hungarian: 188  37  26  28  15   294
        Switzerland:   8  48  32  30   5   123
      Long Beach VA:  51  56  41  42  10   200
```

6.3. NUMERICAL EVALUATION

The experiments are conducted in the mat lab simulation environment where the performance evaluation between the proposed method namely Heart disease prediction using HRS-HMCSVM with our previous work Alpha Rough Set Theory combined with Fuzzy SVM (ARST-FSVM), Fuzzy Rough Set Theory combined with Support Vector Machine (FRS - SVM) and the existing methods namely Coronary Heart Disease prediction using Particle Swarm Optimization Approach (CHD-PSO), Artificial Neural Network based Prediction (ANN) is done. The performance metrics that are considered in this research work for the comparison evaluation are, "Accuracy, Precision, Recall, F-Measure". The performance evaluation are shown and explained in the following sub sections.

6.3.1. Simulation outcome of Accuracy

Accuracy is defined as the proportion of true positives and true negatives among the total number of results obtained. Accuracy is evaluated as,

$$\text{Accuracy} = \frac{(\text{True positive} + \text{True negative})}{(\text{True positive} + \text{True negative} + \text{False positive} + \text{False negative})}$$

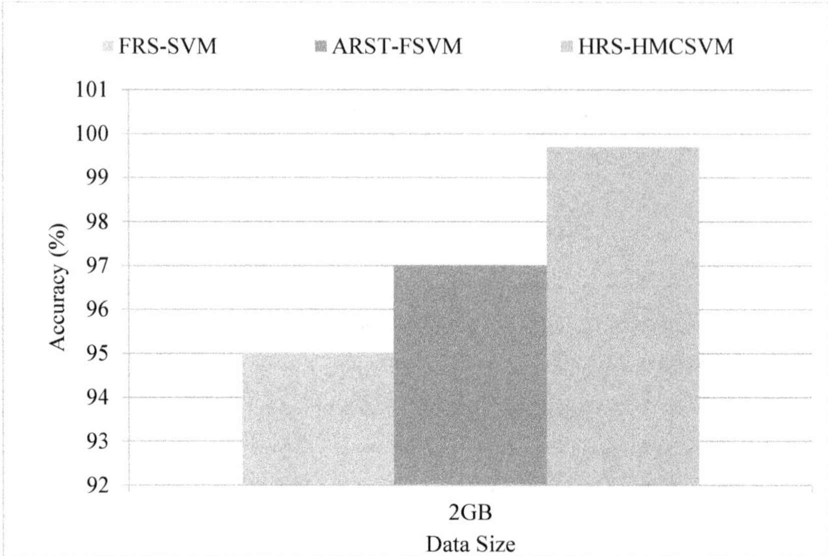

Figure 6.1. Graphical comparison of Accuracy

From the above graph mentioned in (Figure-6.1), it is proved that the proposed method namely HRS-HMCSVM can provide better performance result than the existing research methodologies. From the analytical evaluation of the results, it can be proved that the proposed methodology HRS-HMCSVM is 3% better than ARST-FSVM, 5% better performance than FRS_SVM, 8% better than CHD-PSO, 12% better performance than ANN method.

6.3.2. Simulation outcome of Precision

Precision value is evaluated according to the relevant information at true positive prediction, false positive.

$$\text{Precision} = \frac{\text{True Positive}}{(\text{True Positive} + \text{False Positive})}$$

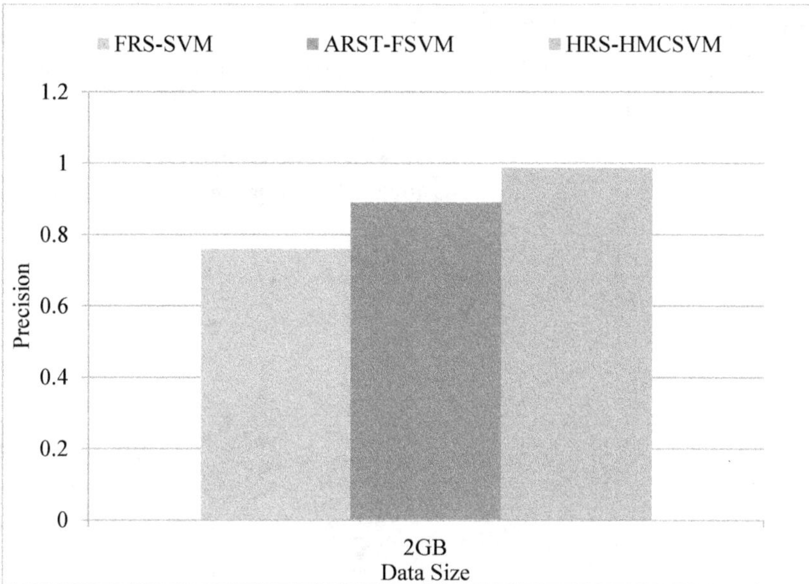

Figure 6.2. Graphical comparison of Precision

From the above graph it is proved that the proposed method namely HRS-HMCSVM can provide better performance result than the existing research methodologies in terms of precision. From the analytical evaluation of the results, it can be proved that the proposed methodology HRS-HMCSVM is 11% better than ARST-FSVM, 30% better outcome than FRS-SVM, 37% better than CHD-PSO, 32% better performance than ANN method.

6.3.3. Simulation outcome of Recall

Recall value is evaluated according to the retrieval of information at true positive prediction, false negative.

$$\text{Recall} = \frac{\text{True Positive}}{(\text{True positive} + \text{False negative})}$$

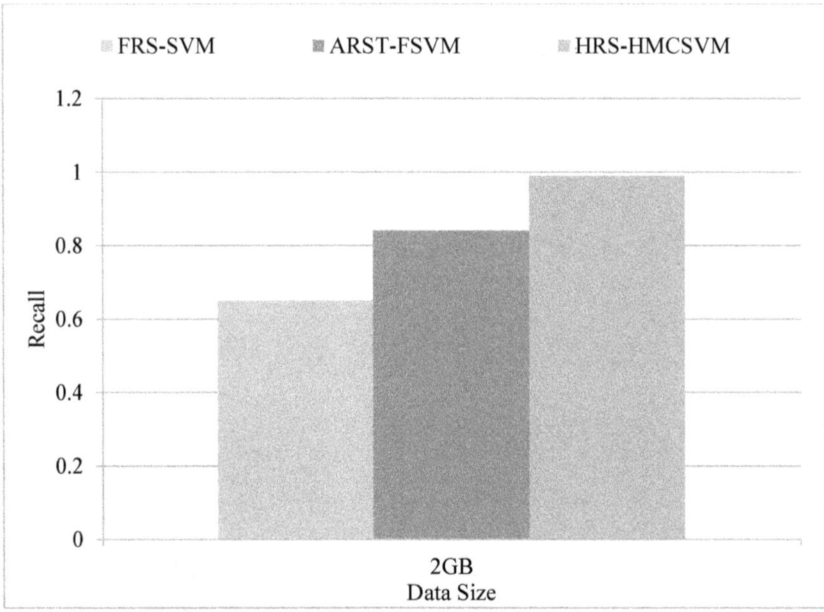

Figure 6.3. Graphical comparison of Recall

From the above graph it is proved that the proposed method namely HRS-HMCSVM can provide better performance result than the existing research methodologies. From the analytical evaluation of the results, it can be proved that the proposed methodology HRS-HMCSVM is 18% better than ARST-FSVM, 52% better result than FRS-SVM, 62% better performance than CHD-PSO, 74% better performance than ANN method

6.3.4. Simulation outcome of F-Measure

The F-Measure computes some average of the information retrieval precision and recall metrics

$$F - \text{Measure} = \frac{2 * \text{precision.recall}}{\text{precision} + \text{recall}}$$

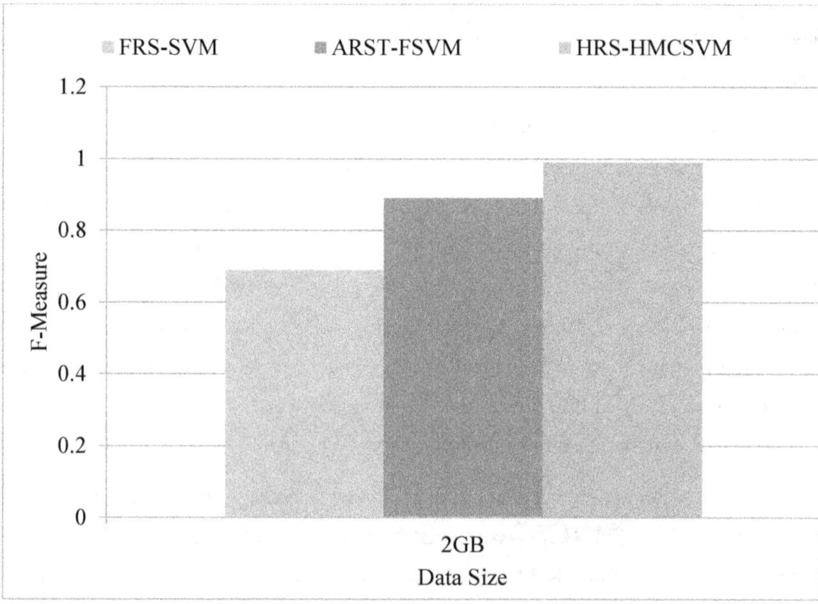

Figure 6.4. Graphical comparison of F-measure

From the above graph it is proved that the proposed method namely HRS-HMCSVM can provide better performance result than the existing research methodologies. From the analytical evaluation of the results, it can be proved that the proposed methodology HRS-HMCSVM is 11% better than ARST-FSVM, 43 % better outcome than FRS-SVM, 57% better than CHD-PSO, 68% better performance than ANN method.

CHAPTER 7

CONCLUSION AND FUTURE WORK

7.1. CONCLUSION

Heart disease has increased quickly by reason of varying lifestyle combined with improper or lack of physical exercise, foretelling and averting the heart diseases at prior stage has turn out to be a significant action as in every year root to death. Plentiful researchers presented in the current work for health disease prediction.

In the first work, initially Pre-processing is done by using K-means clustering Algorithm to make the dataset cleaner, consistent and noise free. Then Feature reduction of the dataset is done by using Fuzzy based rough set theory. The fuzzy rough sets extend the rough set concept through the use of fuzzy equivalence classes. From this reduced feature set, optimal feature selection is done by using Improved Bee Colony approach. Finally, classification of dataset is done by using Support vector machine. The overall evaluation of the proposed research methodology is done by using the Mat lab simulation environment from which it is proved that the proposed work namely NORFS-HDPS can lead to optimal outcome than the existing research techniques.

In the second work introducing the framework namely Heart disease prediction using Alpha Rough Set Theory combined with Fuzzy SVM (ARST-FSVM). In this research method, Modified K-Means clustering algorithm is used for preprocessing the input dataset which would avoid the noisy data present in the database. Then missing data value in the database is handled using normalization technique where NLLS imputation is applied. And then feature dimensionality reduction is done using Alpha rough set theory (α-RST) approach. From those reduced feature set, optimal feature selection in terms of relevancy is done using Hybrid Bee colony algorithm with Glowworm Swarm Optimization (HBC-GSO) approach. Finally heart disease prediction is done using classifier namely fuzzy based SVM. The overall research method ensures that the proposed research technique leads to ensure it can lead to optimal and accurate heart disease diagnosis outcome.

In the third work introducing the Accurate and reliable heart disease prediction with the concern of Risk factors using Hybrid Rough Set-Hybrid Multi Class SVM (HRS-HMCSVM). The proposed research method can optimally predict the heart disease occurrence earlier with increased prediction accuracy. In this research method Hybrid K-Means clustering algorithm is applied to preprocess the dataset. After preprocessing, missing value replacement is done by using imputation methods. And then dimensionality reduction is done by using Hybrid Rough set theory concept which is sent to feature selection module where the optimal features are extracted by using Hybrid Improved Bee Colony with Cuckoo Search Algorithm. Finally, Classification of the dataset is done using Fuzzy SVM approach.

7.2. FUTURE WORK

In future, fuzzy based techniques can be introduced for performing the optimal feature selection i.e., risk factor selection, thus the optimal and accurate outcome can be obtained. A typical FS process includes four fundamental steps called subset generation, subset evaluation, stopping criterion, and result validation. Subset generation is a search procedure, which creates feature subsets for assessment dependent upon some search technique. FS algorithms contain three models: filter models, wrapper models and hybrid models. In forthcoming work would concentrate on the hybridization techniques for FS in heart disease prediction system.

CPSIA information can be obtained
at www.ICGtesting.com
Printed in the USA
LVHW022033070423
743801LV00009B/189

9 782822 194372